a

b

Genetic Improvement for Farmed Ruminants

Luis Orlando Alba Gomez, PhD
Full Professor and Consulting Professor
Discipline: Reproduction and Genetics

Notice

This is a complementary book that is intended to advise and guide those people who deal with Genetic Improvement for Farmed Ruminants. No two patients are the same. Therefore, we cannot be responsible for the actions or treatments administered to animals on farms without our supervision.

Genetic Improvement for Farmed Ruminants

Copyright 2024 by Luis Orlando Alba Gomez
Cover Designer: Igor Alba Espinosa
Copy Editor: Igor Alba Espinosa

All rights reserved

No part of this publication may be reproduced or transmitted in any form or by any means, electronic or mechanical, without the written permission of the publisher.

Printed in the United States of America
Published by: Amazon Kindle Direct Publishing

Dedication

To my children and to all those who collaborated in one way or another in the completion of this work

A Words of Thanks

The many graduate students whom I scientifically guided in serious scientific-student activities, such as Coursework, Diploma Projects or in postgraduate activities such as Specialization and Doctoral Theses, deserve my recognition. The list of graduates would be too long to reproduce here, but many of their names appear in the references at the end of the book.

Preface

This book has been written with the main objective of providing students of Veterinary Medicine, Animal Husbandry and livestock technicians interested in expanding their knowledge of the selection and genetic improvement systems for cattle, buffalo and sheep-goat livestock in tropical conditions. In addition, it serves as a reference material and guide for farmers interested in genetically improving their herds.

Genetic improvement is decisive and inseparable from the production process, and economic efficiency largely depends on it, since animals with higher performance are obtained.

We know that a Genetic Improvement program has to include the calculation of genetic values, using modern methods of Population Genetics, which require a high level of computation, as is the case with behavior and progeny tests. However, we have wanted to simplify the theoretical explanations of General Genetics as much as possible so that they can be understood by the breeder and applied in practice. This work therefore aims to provide the basic knowledge that will enable, at farm level, the appropriate use of the genetic potential of farm ruminants under the conditions of sustainable tropical livestock farming.

I will be very satisfied if these objectives are met.

Índex

Preface	g
Cap. 1 Fundamentals of animal genetic improvement	1
Cap. 2 Selection principles	19
Cap. 3 Selection methods	35
Cap. 4 Mating systems	71
Cap. 5 Selection systems for dairy cattle	110
Cap. 6 Selection systems for beef cattle	128
Cap. 7 Selection systems for buffaloes	150
Cap. 8 Selection systems for sheep and goats	164
Bibliography	173
Glossary	177
Author's review	180

Chapter 1

Fundamentals of animal genetic improvement

Contents:
Introduction. Concepts of Zoogenetics. Principles of population genetics. Inheritance of quantitative traits. Breeder's Functions. Information needed for an effective selection and mating system.

Introduction

Since genetic improvement is based on the Mendelian laws of inheritance that are taught in the subject of General Genetics, this chapter includes, in an abbreviated form, the concepts that underpin population genetics to facilitate the reader's understanding of the contents of the chapters involved with animal genetic selection and improvement and to show how they can be applied to genetic improvement programs in the different species of farm ruminants.

Concepts of Zoogenetics

Inheritance and variability in living beings

Inheritance is understood as the tendency of beings to faithfully reproduce the characteristics of their parents.

Variation is the tendency that is manifested in individuals to differentiate from each other. All organisms will be subject to these two opposing tendencies and the result of their mutual actions depends on the set of characteristics that each one possesses.

Biological inheritance

The only objects that are biologically inherited from parents are the genes contained in the chromosomes of the germ cells from which the body originates once fertilization has occurred.

Gene or gene

It is the hereditary unit present in the chromosomes of the cells. They are responsible for transmitting the characteristics to another generation.

Genotype

It is the total of inheritance, the genetic constitution that an organism receives from its parents. In other words, it is the set of internal properties that make an individual have certain appearance and functions in a given environment.

Phenotype

It is the external manifestation of the characteristics of an individual, its appearance, but also the characteristics that can be measured or perceptible. E.g.: eye color, milk production, etc. The phenotype is nothing more than the sum of the genotype and the environment.

The phenotype of an individual changes continuously, while the genotype is relatively stable throughout its life.

Environment

The environment is the set of factors external to the individual or that exist within it, constituting its living conditions (food, illnesses, climate, housing, treatment it receives, etc.), capable of revealing or enhancing the hereditary power or flow of the animal to express it in the form of greater or lesser production performance (within the limits of its hereditary capacity) depending on whether the peristasis is favorable or adverse for the animal.

The environment includes the natural environment, the artificial environment, food and hygiene, with treatment and functional gymnastics as elements of enhancement of good genotypic qualities.

Because it is good to insist on this, the favorable environment will enhance or allow to manifest itself in its full extent only those qualities that the animal possesses as a wealth inherited from its parents and through them, from its ancestors.

Good genetic material, a good genotype, is therefore essential to achieve good performance on a livestock farm.

Environmental variations

These are caused by environmental influences. They are differences observed in individuals as a result of an action directed at each of them, in the different conditions that surround them.

Forms of reaction of a genotype

This is defined as the differences in the way in which a genotype can react to different environments.

Penetration and expressivity of genes

The appearance of an organism does not always reflect its genetic makeup. In precise terms, two kinds of effects can be noted and measured: penetration, the proportion of genotypes that show an expected phenotype, and expressivity, the degree to which a particular effect is expressed by individuals.

Penetration expresses the interaction of the affected gene or genes with other genes and with the environment. Penetration values equal to 100 percent or 1 correspond to complete penetrance. Lower values are expressions of incomplete penetrance, indicating in this case a form of inheritance, dominant or recessive, of an incomplete or irregular character.

Pleiotropy

Pleiotropy is spoken of when a gene shows influence on more than one character, that is, when a gene modifies or has an effect on more than one character.

Epistasis

It is a type of genetic interaction in which a gene prevents the expression or manifestation of another non-allele gene.

Allelomorphic genes

Schematically we can consider that, in the manifestation of a character, at least two genes with opposite or identical effects are necessarily involved, which are called allelomorphs or alleles.

When the character is made up of a pair of alleles of the same type, the character or ultimately the resulting phenotype is considered homozygous, and when a gene is of one type and the allele of another, it is said that there is heterozygosity, and that the phenotype is heterozygous. Such genes may have different energies, one being more powerful, dominant, and the other weaker, recessive; and then it is understood that the phenotypic manifestation corresponding to the dominant gene will appear whether there is homozygosity or heterozygosity, while the phenotype corresponding to the weak or recessive gene will only manifest itself if the dominant gene is not present, that is, in recessive homozygosity.

Mutation

In genetics and biology, it is an alteration or change in the genetic information (genotype) of a living being (often due to contact with mutagens) and which, therefore, will produce a change in its characteristics, which occurs suddenly and spontaneously, and which can be transmitted or inherited to offspring. This change will be present in a small proportion of the population (variant) or the organism (mutation).

The genetic unit capable of mutating is the gene, which is the unit of hereditary information that forms part of DNA. In multicellular beings, mutations can only be inherited when they affect reproductive cells.

One consequence of mutations can be a genetic disease, however, although in the short term they may seem harmful, in the long-term mutations are essential for our existence. Without mutation there would be no change and without change life could not evolve.

Since a mutation is any change in the nucleotide sequence of DNA, if the mutation affects a single gene, it is called a genetic mutation, if it affects the structure of one or more chromosomes, it is called a chromosomal mutation, and when one or more mutations cause alterations in the entire genome, they are called genomic mutations.

Genetic recombination

This is the process by which meiosis generates combinations of alleles from different loci that differ from the combinations found in the parents.

Loci located on different chromosomes are freely recombined, while those found on the same chromosome are recombined by the crossing of homologous chromosomes. The gametic conjugation that occurs during fertilization promotes heterozygosity and gives an opportunity for recombination.

Migration

In a broad sense, it is the movement of an organism or group of organisms from one location to another. In population genetics, the process of migration refers to the movement of a population and its assimilation by sexual reproduction into a different population.

Genetic drift

Genetic drift or *genetic drift* is an **evolutionary** force that acts in conjunction with **natural selection** to change the allele frequencies of **species** over time. More briefly, it is the random fluctuation of gene frequencies in a population. Like mutation, it causes small changes that accumulate over time and tend to increase genetic differentiation. Although it occurs in all populations, genetic drift is most evident in small plant populations.

Multifactorial or polygenic inheritance

Polygenic inheritance differs from the classical Mendelian scheme in that the full range of variation is covered by graded series in which the parents constitute extremes. Only the averages in the populations are considered and not the individual values.

The averages reflect factors such as dominance, epistasis, cytoplasmic influence, interactions between genes, gene products and interactions with the environment.

Population genetics applies the methods of mathematical statistics, analyzing the structure of breeding units at a given time, as well as the changes that may occur, i.e., the study of population dynamics. For these reasons, polygenic inheritance is a statistical concept.

Because most of the traits of domestic plants and animals that have practical importance (including height, weight, etc.) depend on polygenic inheritance, greater attention has been paid to this principle. It is estimated that 80 % of all practical studies involve quantitative inheritance.

As with other examples of quantitative inheritance, environmental influence is the most confounding factor in the analysis and should be controlled as much as possible. The environment can produce results like those introduced by genes with respect to size differences between large and small varieties.

Animals that grow under unfavorable conditions (parasitized and poorly nourished) will be smaller than others of the same genotype that are in a more suitable environment. Even minor environmental variations can affect the expression of quantitative traits.

For all the above reasons, environmental influence should be controlled as much as possible in any livestock experimental design.

Linkage and crossing over

In each pair of homologous chromosomes there is an enormous quantity of alleles, and this means that the characteristics or phenotypes corresponding to these alleles of the same pair of homologous chromosomes have to be transmitted simultaneously to the offspring, since one of the chromosomes, with its series of genes, passes from the father to the offspring, as another passes from the mother, and when both are united in the child, the different characteristics or phenotypes governed by the corresponding alleles will arise.

This inheritance, simultaneous or in block, is called *factorial linkage*. This means that, if in the same chromosome there was the gene causing a good quality and at the same time the gene causing the black color, and in the homologous chromosome the genes alleles for bad quality and for white color, it would be enough to see the color of the offspring to know if it had good or bad qualities in a certain sense.

Although not in such a simple way, knowledge of the factors or genes that present linkage is of great interest in Zoogenetics. However, this block inheritance, this factorial linkage, sometimes suffers exceptions due to chromosomal *crossing over*, which causes an exchange of segments between the two homologous chromosomes before their separation, that is, a piece or two of one of the homologous chromosomes takes its place in the homologous and vice versa.

Principles of population genetics

Concept of population

A population is a group or set of individuals that share common traits or characteristics.

Populations are characterized by:

a) **Genetic constitution:** It is given by the set of genes that belong to each population and that distinguish one population from another.

b) **Immortality:** The population is immortal because if the individuals that compose it leave descendants, the genotype of the same is not lost, but is transmitted from generation to generation, even if the individuals of each generation die.

c) **Generation interval:** This is the average time that elapses between corresponding stages of the life cycle in successive generations. This interval varies according to the species: 5 years in cattle and 25 years in humans. It also depends on the conditions of exploitation, breeding technique, etc.

d) **Parental and filial generation:** The parental generation is the one that is taken as a basis for initiating a genetic study.

e) **The population:** That originates from the reproduction of the parental generation (parents or relatives) and that is made up of all the descendants is called the filial generation (or the children).

Genotypic frequency and gene frequency

Genotypic frequency is the frequency of a particular genotype in the population, being its proportion or percentage in individuals. The sum of the frequencies of all genotypes together must be unity or 100 %.

The genetic constitution of a population, referring to the genes it carries, is described by means of the arrangement of *gene frequencies*, that is, by the specification of the alleles present in each locus and the numbers or proportions of the different alleles in each locus.

Inheritance of quantitative traits

The traits of greatest economic importance in the breeding of domestic animals are traits determined by the action of many genes located in many loci, that is, they present the so-called polygenic or multifactorial inheritance. Examples of these traits are milk production, fat production, % of fat, growth rate, egg production, wool, etc.

The inheritance of quantitative traits is an extension of Mendelian genetics, resting entirely on Mendelian principles as a basis.

Quantitative traits are characterized by: being governed by genes at many loci; genes are of minor effect; they have continuous variability; the type of gene action is fundamentally additive.

The study methods used in the inheritance of quantitative traits will be based on the observable properties of animal populations, such as means, variances and covariance's.

Phenotypic variance

The phenotypic expression of a trait such as milk production at 305 days of a cow in first lactation is determined by two main components, the genotype (G) and the environment (E), that the milk production of a cow will depend on the genes that she has for that trait and the environment (climate, management, etc.), so we can say that:

$$P = G + E$$

Where: **P** = phenotype

Therefore, each animal in the population has a genotypic value and an environmental value for each character.

The study of the inheritance of quantitative characters is based on the variability of the characters in the population, so in a population of animals where each one has a certain phenotypic value for each character, the phenotypic variability of the character in the population is given by the variance formula.

In practice, this decomposition of the total phenotypic variability into genetic and environmental is done through variance analysis.

Concept of the heritability coefficient (h^2)

Heritability is the most important parameter in Population Genetics, and it tells us what part of the total variability is due to additive genetic variability and is symbolized as h^2; we can also define h^2 as the part of the phenotypic differences between individuals due to genetic differences.

Heritability also expresses the degree of correspondence that exists between the phenotypic and genetic value of an individual, remembering that the square root of $h^2 = h$ and that **h** is the correlation that exists between the genotype and the phenotype, therefore, as this correlation increases, so does heritability and there is a greater correspondence between the phenotype of an individual and its genotype.

It can then be concluded that selection tends to reduce h^2, since it decreases genetic variability, as well as inbreeding. Uniformity in environmental conditions will reduce environmental variability and therefore increase heritability.

The values of the heritability coefficient fluctuate between 0 % and 100 % or between 0 and 1, depending on the scale used.

In the bovine species, values below 0.2 are classified as low, those ranging from 20 to 40 are medium coefficients and those above 40 are considered high.

Breeder's Functions

In Animal Science, the term *breeder* is used to designate the person who is in charge, or by profession, of breeding animals, which includes caring for and feeding them.

In Genetics, the breeder takes care of reproduction and selection in order to improve the population's genetic background and, consequently, is a breeder. In this section, both terms will be used as synonyms.

The raw material with which the breeder must work is a difference in genes, or variations in individuals due to differences in genes. The breeder cannot create new genes but must work with the genetic variation that already exists in his animals. Genetic variation is the result of gene mutations that have occurred during the production of many new generations of animals. These mutations, together with selection, have made some animals more suitable for a particular purpose or a particular environment.

The breeder is now more interested in producing highly efficient producing animals for a particular purpose, e.g. developing a herd that gives the most milk per animal with the least amount of feed consumed or raising the efficiency of beef production and, in addition, increasing the quality of the carcass. In other words, the problem today is not one of developing new and good breeds, but of improving existing ones, or of combining some of them in some way to take advantage of the advantages of heterosis.

Of course, new breeds have been developed in the world, but their superiority over older and more popular breeds has yet to be demonstrated. However, some of these new breeds have been shown to possess different desirable genes.

The role of the breeder, then, is to identify those animals that possess desirable genes or combinations of genes and to concentrate as many of these genes in his herd as possible.

In trying to find the superior animals, the breeder may be puzzled by environmental effects and by the different modes of gene action and interaction. He must compare the performance of animals raised in the same or similar environment to avoid deviations from environmental influences.

Selection of superior individuals should be based on information collected in pedigree records, phenotypic superiority, and progeny testing, if available. His breeding program will be effective if the selected traits have been accurately measured and are highly heritable, indicating that additive action is the cause of most of the genetic variation.

If non additive gene action is the most important genetic influence on the traits he plans to select, his breeding program will first have to include the development of inbred lines. These will then have to be tested in non-inbred matings to identify those with superior ability to take advantage of the effects of heterosis.

Information needed for an effective selection and mating system

In developing a breeding program, the breeder must first decide which traits are most important to select for from an economic standpoint. His decision will depend on the species of farm animals he is working with, the feeding program he intends to use, the type of product he intends to market, and the price of those products.

In most cases, the breeder will limit the number of traits to be selected for in order to include these traits in a single index. The weight the breeder will give to each trait in the index will depend on the heritability of that trait, its relative economic value, and the genetic correlation of that trait with other traits of economic importance. Examples of index formulas are given in the appropriate chapters for each farm ruminant species discussed.

Next, the breeder must become acquainted with the methods that have been developed to make accurate measurements and how to record them; In this way, the breeder can more satisfactorily distinguish between genetic and environmental effects on the animals in the prospective breeding and on the generations during the breeding program.

Actual measurements of traits, weight, milk yield, or percentage of lean meat, should be performed and not estimated.

The use of correction factors to adjust the records of all animals in the herd to a comparable age, to the same age of the maternal basis, for sex, and other variables, will allow the breeder to make more accurate comparisons, where applicable.

Accuracy in selecting genetically superior animals for breeding purposes, and in evaluating the progress of the breeding program, will be increased if the breeder keeps well-written, detailed records.

Another aspect that the breeder needs to know in order to plan his program is which type of gene action, additive or non-additive, has the greatest influence on each trait of economic importance. Additive gene action is indicated when the heritability of the trait is high, as measured by the similarity between the parents and their offspring, and when crossbreeding results in an average F_1 that is closely approximated to the average of its parents.

Additive gene action is also indicated, but not yet proven, when sexual differences for a trait are large. When additive gene action is more influential, mass selection (mating the best for the best) will be more effective. Non-additive gene action is indicated when the heritability of a trait is low, when inbreeding has had detrimental effects, and when gene refreshing by crossbreeding has had beneficial effects. Non-additive gene action is also indicated when the average of individual F_1 differs from the average of the two parental groups (heterosis).

When non additive gene action has the greatest influence on a trait, the greatest improvement in performance will be achieved by crossing with strains or lines of known combining ability. The breeder may wish to produce and select for several different traits of which some are affected by additive and non-additive gene action.

The procedure recommended here might be to form pure lines or strains by selecting for those traits that are highly heritable; then to cross those lines or strains to improve those traits that show heterosis.

The breeder must also know whether genetic correlations are important between the different traits selected and whether these correlations are positive or negative. The breeder can make the plan more effective if he can also determine whether genetic-environmental interactions influence the traits he wishes to select.

The modern breeder must combine the practical knowledge of the empirical with the scientific knowledge of the geneticist, without neglecting either of them. To his scientific background he must incorporate a perfect command of the morphological and physiological characteristics of animals, of their rational feeding, of the process of their reproduction and, what is very important, of the history of the breed to which the animals belong, on which he works to improve them; that is, of the breeds that gave rise to them and of the different phases they have passed through until reaching their present state.

Chapter 2

Principles of Selection

Contents:
Introduction. Natural selection. Artificial selection. Importance of the environment in selection and improvement. Relationship between environmental variance and genotype. Response to selection. Selection intensity. Selection index. Factors that determine biological health. Heredopathology.

Introduction

Selection can be defined as a process in which certain individuals in a population are preferred over others for the production of the next generation. Selection is natural when natural forces intervene, and artificial when it is due to the efforts of man.

Through selection, new genes are not created. Under the pressure of selection there is a tendency to reduce the frequency of undesirable genes, and to increase the frequency of more desirable genes. Thus, the main genetic defect of selection is to change the arrangement of gene frequencies and also to increase the homozygosity of desirable genes in the population.

Natural Selection

In nature the main force responsible for selection is the ability to survive in a particular environment.

Natural selection is a very complicated process, and numerous factors determine the proportion of individuals that will reproduce.

Among these factors are differences in the mortality of individuals in the population, especially at early ages; differences in the length of the period of sexual activity; the degree of sexual activity itself and differences in the degree of fertility of individuals in the population.

Weak, poorly endowed or sick animals are chosen by predators for consumption, and this is a form of natural selection.

It is interesting to note that in animals in the wild and even in those domesticated to a certain extent, there is a tendency to eliminate defective or harmful genes that have arisen because of mutations.

Artificial Selection

Artificial selection is that which is practiced by man. In this way, man determines which animals will be used to produce subsequent offspring.

The selection that results from the breeder's action in choosing the parents produces changes in the gene frequency by separating the adult individuals of the paternal generation into two groups, the selected and the discarded, groups that differ in their gene frequencies.

It has been proven that artificial selection has been effective, in many cases, in achieving well-defined differences between breeds and types within farm animal species, both to modify some qualitative and quantitative traits.

Importance of the environment in selection and improvement

One of the biggest mistakes that has been made, almost everywhere, is to try to implement an animal improvement program without taking into account the conditions not only of the climate, but also of agricultural improvement and the economic-social environment.

The rancher and also the administrative authorities, in their eagerness to move more quickly, ignore the basic principles of acclimatization and adaptation of imported animals.

The adaptation of dairy or meat animals and their improvement process cannot be separated from agricultural improvement, the production of better-quality fodder and the possibility of feeding the animals adequately throughout the year.

In parallel with the importation of animals from temperate climates, it is necessary to create ecological conditions that promote environmental well-being, by planting leafy trees in grazing areas and dairy farms, to protect them from strong solar radiation and heat.

The breeding policy in the tropics is a very complex matter, because it depends on many factors that must be taken into consideration, such as: the development of agriculture, the possibility of using crops for animal feed, the social and economic living conditions of the farmers, the facilities for valorizing milk at a level compatible with the higher maintenance costs. Once all these facets of the problem have been assessed, the conclusion is reached that the best cow is often not the one that produces the most milk, but the one that best adapts to all the requirements under which it will necessarily have to be exploited.

The genetic improvement program should not be limited to knowing which European breeds are the best producers of milk or meat, but to creating the conditions for preserving them better from the inclemency of the tropical climate and establishing a nutritional program appropriate to the susceptibilities of their digestive system and their nutritional needs in accordance with the functions for which their digestive system is intended.

If these aspects are not met, imported breeds do not adapt properly because they fail in the environmental resistance mechanisms included in the ecological law of *Limiting Factors*.

This law refers to *the limiting effect of the excess or deficit of any environmental factor on performance. Thus, the possibility of subsistence or development and the performance of an organism are conditioned by the reduced presence below the minimum critical level or exceeding the maximum tolerance level of an environmental factor, which is called the "limiting factor"*.

The warm-humid climate of the tropics, with two seasons of irregular rainfall, with maximum air temperatures of 30-35 degrees Celsius, high relative humidity and high solar radiation, the abundance of external and internal parasites, tropical diseases, as well as prolonged periods of drought, with the consequent food shortage, constitute the main limiting factors for livestock. Add to this the deep-rooted habits of livestock farmers of not producing food for their animals, or preserving it for times of food shortage.

Fortunately, there is the possibility of compensation to reduce the effect of any limiting factor. Thus, it has been shown that the use of an appropriate feed in dairy cattle can substantially reduce the harmful effect of high tropical temperatures, up to certain ranges.

It can be deduced then that, as a logical and important result for the breeding of domestic animals, it is evident that each form of artificial selection must be simultaneously conditioned by the improvement of environmental conditions.

Relationship between environmental variance and genotype

The factors or genes that affect continuous variation are many, and they do so in a cumulative manner; for example, if one bull has a very high weight and another a very low weight, the genetic difference between them lies in the fact that the high-weight bull was determined by many genes that control this characteristic and that give rise to a product that increases weight; on the contrary, the low-weight bull was also produced by many genes that control this weight, allelic genes of the high-weight ones that result in a lower weight increase.

If, for example, seven pairs of genes control the weight of bulls in a given breed, the genotypes for high and low weight would be:

| AABBccDDEEFFGG | (high weight) |
| aabbCCddeeffgg | (low weight) |

Capital letters are alleles for high weight and lowercase letters for low weight.

Each allele contributes equally in a certain amount to the increase of the trait, starting from a minimum value given by the rest of the genotype.

The environment affects the phenotype produced by these genes, so that many times this phenotype does not correspond to the genotype that determines it.

In our example, the high weight genotype results in a phenotype of 800 kg, which we can consider as that which occurs in an average environment. But if other individuals with this same genotype were raised in a nutrient-poor environment, this would influence the amount of the product for the weight controlled by their genes, and the real weight would not be 800 kg, but, for example, 600 kg. On the other hand, if the environment is favorable, the product in question increases, and the weight would be 900 kg instead of 800 kg.

In summary, the phenotype of all continuously varying traits is defined by a genetic part (genotype) and by a part largely determined by the environment where the individual developed.

The improvement of the traits exploited by man in plants and animals presents this type of continuous variation; therefore, the improvement of the environment where they are raised is of vital importance, since with this we will achieve the expression in the phenotype of the best genotypes for their selection.

In the crossings of individuals that differ in some continuously varying trait, the genes that control this are segregated independently and recombine with each other, following the principles discovered by Mendel.

The fact that the phenomena of dominance and recessivity or the Mendelian proportions in the F_2 are not observed in these crosses, is due to the peculiar cumulative effect that these genes have. Most continuously varying traits exhibit this peculiar mode of inheritance.

Response to selection

In general, the purpose of a selection program in an animal population is to select as parents of the next generation those individuals whose offspring, as a group, have the highest genetic merit for the trait or traits in question.

This is equivalent to selecting as parents of the next generation those whose additive genetic merit is the highest. If this is true, the population mean will change from one generation to the next. This is the *response to selection*, which is symbolized by **R** and is defined as the difference between the phenotypic mean of the offspring of the individuals selected as parents and the mean of the original population; the value obtained is called the *selection differential* and is symbolized by **S**.

In other words, the change produced by selection that matters most is that of the population mean. This change is the *selection response*.

The mean of the applied selection is the average superiority of the selected parents and is called the *selection differential*.

The coefficient of the response on the selection differential is equal to the heritability and the response is given by means of:

$$R = h_2 S$$

The deviation of the progeny from the population mean is, by definition, the reproductive value of the parents and in this way the response is equivalent to the reproductive value of the parents. It is therefore concluded that the expected value of the progeny is given by the expression:

$$R = h_2 S$$

Selection differential

The amount of selection pressure applied to a particular trait is known as the *selection differential*. This *differential* is the average difference between the herd average and the average of the individuals within the herd that are retained for breeding purposes.

We will use the back fat thickness of a pig as an example: The average fat thickness of a group of pigs was 37.5 mm at 100 kg body mass.

From this group, boars and sows, those that averaged 28.5 mm fat thickness at 100 kg were selected. The selection differential is the difference between the average of all pigs in that group (37.5) and the average of the individuals retained for breeding purposes (fat thickness of sows plus fat thickness of boars divided by two), or 9.0 mm.

In general, the greater the selection differential, the greater the progress that can be expected by making the selection.

A number of factors can affect the value of the selection differential. These include the number of animals that can be culled in the selection process as breeding stock, or the number of animals needed to maintain for replacement purposes.

The number of traits selected will tend to reduce the value of the selection differential for any one trait. The reason for this is that an animal that is excellent at one trait may be mediocre at another or several others.

In other words, it is much more difficult to find an individual that is excellent at several traits than one that is excellent at only one. For this reason, it is advisable not to select for too many traits at the same time.

Selection intensity

The standard deviation, which is the measure of variability, is a property of the character of the population and provides the units with which the response is expressed, that is, so many kilograms, so many millimeters, so many mushrooms, etc.

The response to selection can be generalized if both the response and the selection differential are expressed in terms of the standard deviation. phenotypic.

Then: $\boxed{\dfrac{R}{aP}}$ It is a generalized measure of response, by which we can compare different traits and different populations to carry out selection. The "*standardized*" selection differential is called the selection intensity, and is symbolized by **i**.

The intensity of selection, **i**, depends solely on the proportion of the population included in the selected group and can be determined by means of the normal distribution tables, provided that the distribution of the phenotypic values is normal.

Selection index

To do this, the point gain or total score method is used, which consists of selecting all the traits simultaneously, by using the net merit index, constructed by adding, in a single figure, the credits and penalties given to each animal, according to the degree of its superiority or inferiority in each trait. This procedure is called the selection index method.

Factors that condition biological health

Healthy animal

To understand what the inheritance of health is, we have to define what a healthy animal is.

A healthy animal is one that from birth shows signs of having the conditions to overcome the adverse factors of the natural environment. It shows a good physique at birth and without defects. It grows at a pace, achieves perfect development and reproduces properly.

This means that precocity, physical vigor, resistance to disease, fertility and longevity are some of the most important factors that determine biological health. Consequently, the inheritance of health is the capacity of animals to transmit the aforementioned factors to their descendants.

Hereditary health assessment by phenotype

Hereditary health assessment by phenotype includes phenotypic testing of the breeder for favorable or unfavorable traits of hereditary origin.

It should not be forgotten that most of the hereditary defects known to us are recessive. This means that an apparently healthy animal may be the carrier of an unfavorable hereditary trait.

Hereditary health assessment by ancestors

The second possibility of assessing the health of a breeder is that carried out by virtue of its ancestors and relatives. Selection by pedigree or genealogy has become very important in achieving the desired conformation and performance.

This type of health assessment can be considered useful for applying selection to young animals that do not have their own production records. However, it has the disadvantage that the environmental conditions under which the ancestors were evaluated change in relation to those under which the individual is being evaluated.

Assessment of health inherited by offspring

The third term is the assessment of offspring, which is not always possible in older animals due to their duration. However, this method offers the best possibilities for diagnosing hereditary faults and unfavorable (undesirable) dispositions of a breeder.

This is the most precise way to assess the genetic value of an individual, since it studies the offspring of different individuals to determine which group is superior.

Hereditary resistance to diseases

Resistance is the property of the organism to reject or resist infectious diseases and unfavorable environmental conditions. It is conditioned by a series of physiological, biochemical or immunological factors, which in turn are genetically controlled.

Due to the great complexity of resistance, it has been necessary to classify it for evaluation into:

1- Resistance to unfavorable environmental factors

2- Resistance to nutritional deficiencies

3- Resistance to infectious diseases

Resistance to adverse environmental factors

It is evaluated through the adaptation properties, through which the organism receives the ability to survive in certain conditions.

The adaptation possibilities are determined by the genotype of each individual and the possible extent of this capacity at the population level is called genetic homeostasis.

Resistance to nutritional deficiencies

Its existence is known in most species, but especially in domestic birds. Some lines of birds have a greater capacity to tolerate diets deficient in some amino acids.

Resistance to infectious diseases

One of the most important resistance mechanisms is the so-called natural immunity, another resistance mechanism is the cellular defensive reaction of the organism.

It has been shown that it is possible to select based on genetic resistance against certain diseases.

This selection is very difficult to carry out in larger species, because the methods to determine resistance are very complicated and the generation interval is also very long. However, some observations have shown that there is a genetic resistance against mastitis. An increased frequency of mastitis has been found in daughters of affected mothers. The heritability of resistance to this disease has been determined to be between 0.25 and 0.40.

Similar observations have been made indicating genetic resistance against tuberculosis and some protozoan diseases in cattle; against hepatic adenomatosis, parasitosis and gangrene in sheep; against brucellosis, erysipelas and atrophic rhinitis in pigs.

However, except for poultry, genetic improvement of domestic animals by selection for resistance against some diseases is still a remote possibility, due to the practical and economic difficulties involved in carrying it out.

Heredopathology

This is the science that deals with the hygiene of heredity and generally studies the phenomena and laws related to the inheritance of diseases, anomalies, deformations, as well as all constitutional abnormalities and organic weaknesses that animals present at birth or later as a consequence of pathological hereditary factors received from one or both parents.

Lethal and sublethal genes

In all populations, the alleles responsible for causing, in their carriers, more or less expressive defects or causing death are found in certain loci of the chromosomes.

Malformations with a recognized genetic cause are called hereditary defects, unlike phenocopies, which are anomalies due to external disturbances that occur during the course of embryonic development. In this case, the genetic code is normal, but the course of morphogenesis is disturbed.

From the point of view of genetic improvement, the breeder is mainly interested in non-lethal defects that may appear in animals in an expressive or hidden way, and which are reasons for culling.

Non-lethal hereditary defects or factors caused by autosomal recessive inheritance (*incomplete penetrance genes*)

- **Lordosis** - Deviation of the spine downwards.
- **Syphosis** - Upward deviation.
- **Scoliosis** - To one side.
- **Double croup** - Hypertrophy of the croup muscles.
- **Spastic paresis** - Shortening of the Achilles tendon in one of the hind limbs, altering the aplomb.
- **Spasmophilia** - Involuntary spasmodic contracture of the skeletal muscles. Mechanical and electrical hyperexcitability of the NS that creates a predisposition to spasmodic contracture. It resembles tetany.

- **Hermaphroditism** - Intersexual state.
- **White heifer disease** - Hereditary disease associated or not with white skin color and affecting the development of the Mullerian ducts.
- **Gonadal hypoplasia** - Total or partial underdevelopment of the gonads.
- **Cryptorchidism** - Retention of the testicles in the abdominal cavity.
- **Phimosis** - Congenital narrowing of the foreskin that prevents the penis from coming out.
- **Constitutional frigidity** - Decreased or absent sexual libido in the male. Sexual indifference or apathy.
- **Abdominal hernias**
- **Umbilical hernia**
- **Inguinal and scrotal hernia**

Chapter 3

Selection methods

Contents:
Introduction. Evaluating genetic value. Selection based on individuality. Selection based on ancestors. Selection based on collateral relatives. Selection based on offspring. Tandem selection. Selection based on the integrity and functionality of the reproductive system. Animal model using the BLUP methodology. Genomic sciences. Some applications of molecular markers in livestock farming. Predictive value of genomic selection.

Introduction

The phenotypic value of traits is the only way that can be determined directly under existing environmental conditions. When applied to dairy production in cows, for example, the phenotypic value provides a very uncertain assessment of the genotype of the individual animal. This trait is also limited by sex, since it is not manifested in the male. However, it is necessary to calculate the value of the genes that the bull can transmit to its descendants, that is, its value as a breeder

Evaluating genetic value

The determination of the value of a breeding stock is based on the calculation of the average effect of the genes that an individual transmits to its descendants in random matings within the population. In this respect, the age of the animal is not taken into account; but the earlier a male is checked, the better.

The general value of breeding stock is determined by the additive (average) effect of the genes in the combinations in which they can occur within their population.

The special value depends on the modifications that the additive effect of the genes undergoes as a consequence of dominance and epistasis.

Selection based on individuality

This selection is based on the individual's own phenotype. Selection can be made for some traits, such as conformation, growth rate or carcass quality.

Selection based on own phenotype provides good results when heritability is high, although its effect decreases as its value decreases.

The fact that selection based on own phenotype is characteristic of traits with high heritability is based on the fact that in these cases the phenotype reflects the genotype with a high probability and therefore can be transmitted to their descendants.

The greatest disadvantage of selection based on own phenotype is that, often, environmental and genetic effects are difficult to distinguish and for this reason, comparison is necessary for selection purposes under a standard environment.

Selection based on ancestors

Genealogical selection is based on the characteristics of its ancestors (ancestors and collaterals), which are recorded in purebred animals in the pedigree or genealogical album, which can be acquired to analyze the productive behavior of these ancestors in each generation.

This selection, based on ancestors, is carried out to choose from a group of young breeders that have not yet undergone the progeny test, the most outstanding genealogically and morphologically to be used as future breeders.

Similarly, the pedigree is studied when a bull or semen from the same is to be acquired with certain desirable characteristics to mate with females or herds in which it is desired to improve these characteristics in the offspring, such as: milk production, percentage of fat in milk, morphology, etc.

The pedigree is also used to select individuals not related to the female population in order to avoid inbreeding and to favor interlineal or interfamilial heterosis.

In addition, the pedigree allows the grouping of breeders by kinship and the formation of genealogical lines, each of them outstanding in some productive characteristic, which can be used when wanting to improve that characteristic.

The formation of these lines in a country of a certain breed creates the breed structure, makes it more plastic, enables the realization of a more intense and effective selection and fundamentally avoids inbreeding, favoring heterosis with the adequate rotation of the bull lines in the massive use of artificial insemination.

Selection based on collateral relatives

Pedigree study

To know the ancestry of the individual, it is necessary to resort to the genealogical book kept in the breeding centers. This book contains records of all the most important data that attest to the zootechnical value of the animal for dairy or meat production, in relation to the ancestry and descendants of the animal in question.

It is, so to speak, a family tree in which, in addition to the names and direct family kinship, the productions of the females and males are recorded, in the scale of ancestry or descent.

Genealogical books are very important in the improvement of breeds and are organized into breeds or sub-breeds, as is the case of the Dutch-Argentine, Carnation, Indo-Brazilian, etc.

It is a task that must be organized by breeders' associations, so that there can be a sufficiently high number of registrations and that it allows the exchange of data with a view to the selection or choice of the most advisable breeders in each particular case. It is very difficult to establish a new breed without resorting to the genealogical book and without the guarantee of collaboration of several breeders.

When purebred animals are not registered in the purebred books (Herd Book) they lose economic value because their owners do not have any document that accredits their animals as pure and no buyer would risk an investment without a guarantee.

These breed books have served to maintain the racial characteristics since they do not admit animals that do not respond to the prototype of the breed, that have morphological defects, or crossbreeding traits, etc.

All the widely spread breeds have branches in each country to guarantee the racial requirements.

In the official pedigree, the following information appears using acronyms, generally in English:

a) Morphological classification and percentage of that qualification in the breed records of everyone contained in the pedigree and of its offspring.

Example:

Father:

Evaluation	Points
Excellent	≤ 90
Very good	85-89
Good plus	80-84
Good	75-79
Fair	65-74
Poor	> 65

b) Summary of milk and fat production of each bull's daughters in 305 days of lactation according to age or lactation (the total average of those that completed their lactation) and fat percentage. These total averages are also reflected in **B.C.A.** points for milk and fat and the number of daughters that were compared in the progeny test with herd mates (**D.W.H**) or with contemporaries (**C.C**) and the average **B.C.A.** points achieved.

Meaning of these acronyms:

- **B.C.A. (Breed Class Average)** or average of the breed by age or category. It is the average milk and fat production index of the breed for each age or lactation.

- **One B.C.A.** point is equivalent to 100 lb of milk (54.5 kg) and 100 B.C.A. points represent the average milk and fat production for that age or category.

- **D.W.H. (Daughter with Herd mates)** or daughters compared to stablemates.

- **The D.W.H.** are production records of cows in their first lactation (2 years) compared to the production of their herd mates that calved in the same season of the year. These records are expressed in terms of B.C.A. A bull with 200 daughters with + 8 points of B.C.A. means that his offspring improve the breed average by 8 points in fat or milk.

- **C.C. (Comparison with Contemporary)** or comparison with contemporaries is a widely used method of progeny testing based on the comparison of the daughters of a bull with contemporary daughters of other bulls that have calved in the same season of the year and under equal conditions.

- **W. (Weighing)** the number of daughters and contemporaries that entered the test is called Weighing or (effective daughters) to use a factor that weights the participation of the bull's daughters and contemporaries. The higher this number is, the more certain the results are.

c) Awards from exhibitions or fairs obtained by the animal or its offspring such as: **All Canadian**, **Reserve All Canadian** and **Honorable Mention**.

- **Likewise,** the recognition of the *Honor List*, which corresponds to cows that have had productions of more than 100,000 lbs of milk.

- **Superior Type**: awarded to the bull with daughters that exceed the average of the type (morphology of the breed).

- Extra Class: When the two previous awards are obtained for two consecutive years.

- In the USA, the Extra Class will be awarded the Gold Medal and the Silver Medal for Production and Type will be awarded, which are equivalent to the Superior Production and Superior Type awards used in Canada.

d) The production records of the females, their lifetime production and the average of their B.C.A. indices. in these lactations:

- **2y-3y:** means 2 years-3 years, that is, 2nd and 3rd lactation.

- **3x:** means three milkings, unless the pedigree indicates that only two milkings were performed.

The pedigree must ensure that the productive improvement reflected by the data is progressive, that is, the parents must have higher values than the grandparents and these than their ancestors.

Disadvantages of the pedigree

The disadvantages of the pedigree can be indicated as follows:

a) The incomplete heritability of the characters.

b) The different possibilities of combination resulting from Mendelian segregation in characters with polygenic inheritance.

c) The production records of the ancestors may be several years old and have been obtained in environmental conditions different from those of the individual being evaluated.

If inheritance were totally additive and $h^2 = 1$, then from a statistical point of view each parent would be responsible for 25 % of the variation in the offspring and the remaining 50 % should be attributed to Mendelian segregation.

This is the maximum information that can be obtained with the pedigree, considering both parents and for each ancestor, it is reduced by half and so on, so the fundamental weight should be given to the most recent ancestors and beyond the third or fourth generation it should not be considered since it would have very little influence.

Despite these considerations, the pedigree can be used to decide when two or more animals are very similar in their behavior, but one has a more desirable pedigree than the other.

Pedigree information is also very useful when animals are selected at a young age and their production is not known in identifying superior families.

Selection based on offspring

This method of selecting bulls is based on the female offspring of the same bull, which is why it is called *progeny testing*.

It is considered the most reliable and accurate method for evaluating breeding stock for racial and productive improvement. The performance and quality of the offspring provide the final answer on the use of an animal as a breeder.

Progeny tests are very useful for determining traits that are expressed only in one sex, such as milk production, egg production, and they are also useful for measuring those traits that cannot be measured in the living animal, such as carcass characteristics.

There are several methods of progeny testing, but we will refer only to the most widely used and well-known.

Mother-daughter comparison

The Holstein-Friesian Association of America (1966) selects bulls by making comparisons between the production of daughters and mothers, based on equivalent daily milkings at adult age, requiring the following requirements:

a) No less than 10 pairs of daughters-mothers, with no less than 15 controlled lactations of the daughters.

b) The average fat percentage of daughters must be at least 3.4 %.

c) The average production of daughters must not be less than that of the breed (6 251.4 kg of milk and 231.0 kg of fat) and must exceed the *expectancy* established in advance, according to the number of daughter-mother pairs in variable amounts. This expectancy is the midpoint between the breed average and the average of the mothers.

Contemporary Comparison (C.C.)

In the evaluation of the progeny test, milk production is affected by environmental differences from one herd to another by an estimate of 80 to 90 %.

To overcome the effect of this variation, the C.C. method was developed in which the first lactation of the daughters of a bull is compared with the daughters of other bulls of the same herd and time.

The *accuracy* or *precision* of the comparison depends mainly on the number of effective daughters. The greater the number of these and the more tests performed, the greater the merit of the evaluation.

The composition and structure of the milk are also considered when making the final selection.

Notes:

1- Each herd and each year is treated separately.

2- The production of contemporaries is subtracted from the production of daughters of the bulls evaluated to give the average difference. When there are no contemporaries the record of daughters is excluded from the calculation.

3- For correct emphasis each difference must be weighted according to the number of daughters and contemporaries on which it is based.

4- The total weighted difference is divided by the total effective daughters to give the CC result. A refinement of the method is the use of "weighting factors" or effective daughters.

The weighting given to each record is calculated by the following formula:

$$\frac{\text{No. daughters} \times \text{No. contemporaneous}}{\text{No. daughters} + \text{No. contemporaneous}}$$

Example:

1	daughters with	3	contemporaneous	=	0,7	effectives
2	daughters with	2	contemporaneous	=	1,0	effectives
3	daughters with	2	contemporaneous	=	1,2	effectives
3	daughters with	5	contemporaneous	=	1,9	effectives

This means that two daughters and two contemporaries provide the same amount of information as one daughter at a progeny testing station, when conditions are perfectly controlled.

In Canada, a minimum of 20 effective daughters is required for the results of the contemporary comparison to be officially published.

A bull with a rating of +2 is 2% above the breed average, and his daughters are expected to produce 2 % (or two B.C.A. points) above that average as well. One B.C.A. point is equivalent to 100 pounds of milk in the Holstein breed and somewhat less in other dairy breeds.

According to collateral relatives

Collateral relatives are those who are not directly related to an individual, such as his ancestors and progeny, that is, his brothers, uncles, nephews, cousins, of a given animal.

The most commonly used collateral relatives are the families of brothers and half-brothers, as they can provide very valuable information on the value of an individual as a breeder, especially when the heritability of the trait is low and there are numerous groups of brothers.

When a boar has sired several litters with different sows, information can be obtained on:

1- The performance of his own sons.

2- The group of brothers of his father and mother to which he belongs.

3- The groups that are half-brothers of him.

In all family selection, a cause of error must be taken into account as a consequence of the fact that the relatives can live in different environmental conditions

Tandem Selection

First, one trait is selected until it is improved, then for a second trait, until finally each trait has been improved to a desired level.

According to independent levels

In this, a certain level of merit is established for each trait and all individuals below the level are discarded, regardless of superiority or inferiority in the other traits.

Selection based on the integrity and functionality of the reproductive system

An important aspect to take into account when incorporating an animal into the reproductive program is to evaluate the anatomical and functional integrity of its reproductive system.

It is useless for an animal to have an excellent genotype and external conformation if its genital system presents defect that limit or prevent fertility, or is a carrier of undesirable genes. This evaluation must be carried out by a veterinarian knowledgeable in gynecology or veterinary andrology.

Selection of the female

The evaluation requires an external and internal clinical examination. The vulva will be inspected for proportional size, persistence of the hymen or any other defect. A vaginal examination will be done to check its length and permeability.

For the inspection of the internal genital apparatus, a rectal examination will be carried out in which the size, shape and consistency of the cervix, uterine horns, tubes and ovaries will be evaluated. This is done in order to detect possible alterations in the development of these organs, of a congenital or hereditary nature.

The anatomical characteristics of the reproductive apparatus of all bovine breeds of the *Bos taurus* species are very similar to those of *Bos indicus*, except for the ovaries and cervix.

The lack of knowledge of the particularities of the size and shape of the ovaries of Zebu cattle and their crossbreds can lead to diagnostic errors and to discard animals for being presumably hypoplastic, or suffering from ovaritis or ovarian sclerosis.

In a study carried out over several years, this author characterized the size and shape of the ovaries and cervix of Zebu females and their crossbreds. It was found that in heifers and commercial Zebu cows there are three types of ovaries that differ in size and shape and can be as small as a pea (0.8 cm) and as large as a corn cob (5-5.5 cm).

It was particularly curious that these three types of ovaries were also observed in heifers, although the large and bulging ovary of these was smaller than that of cows. On the other hand, the small ovary was found in both heifers and cows.

It should be noted that no degree of association was found between the size and shape of the ovaries and reproductive behavior, body mass or age.

This means that the types of ovaries were found in both prepubescent heifers and old cows, recently calved, pregnant, etc., so this finding should be considered as an anatomical characteristic of this *Bos indicus* subspecies.

In heifers and cows of the Cuban Zebu breed, a higher frequency of the small ovary type was observed, but the large and dented ovary type, characteristic of the crossbred Zebu, was not found.

The observation of crossbred heifers in a backward cross ¾ Zebu x ¼ Brown Swiss showed that in this crossbreeding the three types of ovaries inherited from the Zebu parents were present. In the absorbing Holstein x Zebu cross (F_1), this same finding was also true in 13 % of the cows, but not in the heifers.

In both crosses the percentage of hypertrophied and deformed cervices was relatively high, which indicates that the gonadal and cervical morphological traits of Zebu cattle are transmitted through inheritance and apparently have a dominant character.

As the absorbing cross tended towards homozygosity with a predominance of *Bos taurus* genes, the frequency of appearance of the three types of ovaries, mainly the large and dented one, decreased until almost disappearing in the second filial generation or F_2, but the small ovary type remained with a high frequency. However, the type of deformed cervix typical of Zebu cattle tended to disappear with the homozygosity of *Bos taurus*.

Selection of the male

The clinical examination of the reproductive system is the most effective and reliable procedure to evaluate the reproductive aptitude of a breeding male and is carried out with two main purposes:

a) Select the animal as a future breeder.
b) Carry out the andrological diagnosis of an animal that presents reproductive disorders. These actions are very important since a breeding male is worth what he is capable of contributing in terms of the production of offspring.

The first clinical examination that is carried out on a bull to evaluate it as a future breeder does not have to be complete, but rather limited to the external examination of the testicles, mainly, if they are contained in the scrotal sac, their consistency and their size.

At the age of 24 to 26 months, a second clinical examination should be performed, which includes a general examination, examination of the testicles, internal examination of the accessory sexual glands, and measurement of libido and reaction time.

The clinical examination of the reproductive system performed on an adult male intended for natural mating with infertility problems or low fertility should begin with the measurement of libido and reaction time. That is, evaluating his performance during copulation.

Based on this evaluation, the andrologist should decide whether it is worth continuing with the rest of the examinations or recommend eliminating the animal as a breeder.

Dynamics of testicular development

It has been observed that the testicles of bulls describe an appreciable dynamic of development in the stage of body growth that progressively decreases as the animal becomes an adult, but this process of gonadal growth does not have the same dynamics in all breeds.

This can be seen more clearly when comparing the testimetric values of bulls of different breeds in Tables 3-1 to 3-5, which describe the dynamics of testicular development at different ages.

In studies carried out in Cuba, it was found that Brown Swiss bulls had a more dynamic development than Holsteins up to the age of 13-16 months; from that age onwards, Holstein bulls had a more intense testicular dynamism and surpassed the testimetric values of Brown Swiss bulls (Tables 3-1 and 3-2).

In crossbred bulls ¾ Holstein x ¼ Zebu, a greater dynamism in testicular development was observed at the ages of 6-11 and 12-17 months. Development remained slow until the age of 36-41 months and decreased at 42 months.

One of the characteristics of these bulls is the poor development of the length of the testicles at the age of eight to eleven months, compared to the width and thickness, which gives the testicles a rather oval shape (Table 3-3).

In the ⅝ Holstein x ⅜ Zebu bulls, the greatest testicular dynamics are observed between six and 17 months. As in the ¾ Holstein x ¼ Zebu bulls, the testicles have little development in length (Table 3-4).

In *Bos indicus* bulls, the IVT was 2.5 times lower than in *Bos taurus* bulls at 12 months of age and 180 points lower at 24 months. However, the testicular volume index values were similar when all bulls reached 36 months of age.

These results indicate the need for breeders to be familiar with the dynamics of testicular development in the breed of bulls that are going to be selected for testicular size, mainly at the ages of 12, 24 and 36 months, and not be guided by generalizations that may be misleading.

Below are five tables with the values of the biometry of the right testicle of *Bos taurus* bulls and their crosses with *Bos indicus*, which show the dynamics of gonadal development by age.

Table 3-1 Testicular biometry of Holstein bulls

Age/months	Length	Width	Thickness	TVI
8-12	10,3±1,3	5,8±0,7	5,7±0,7	300±97
23-26	12,9±0,5	7,3±0,2	7,1±0,4	539±56
36-48	13,2±1,3	8,1±0,8	8,1±0,6	717±169

Table 3-2 Testicular biometry of Brown Swiss bulls

Age/months	Length	Width	Thickness	TVI
8-12	11,6±1,4	6,2±0,3	6,2±0,4	401±85
23-26	12,4±1,1	6,7±0,6	6,6±0,5	488±105
36-48	13,0±1,5	7,3±0,5	7,3±0,5	582±123

Table 3-3 Testicular biometry of ¾ Holstein x ¼ zebu

Age/months	Length	Width	Thickness	TVI	SC
6-11	5,9+0,1	5,0+0,1	5,0+0.9	156±8	26,2+0,5
12-17	7,8+0,3	6,3+0,2	6,3+0,2	322±13	33,4+0,5
18-23	8,9+0,5	6,9+0,3	6,8+0,3	428±23	35,2+0,8
30-35	9,2+0,4	7,1+0,2	6,7+0,2	472±21	35,8+0,6
36-41	9,5+0,6	7,2+0,5	7,1+0,5	506±35	36,3+1,4

Table 3-4 Testicular biometry of ⅝ Holstein x ⅜ zebu

Age/months	Length	Width	Thickness	TVI	SC
6-11	5,6+0,1	4,4+0,1	4,4+0,1	121±6	24,0±04
12-17	8,2+0,2	6,2+0,1	6,2+0,1	307±15	30,8±06
18-23	8,4+0,3	6,5+02	6,5+0,2	416±22	31,0±05
30-35	9,3+0,2	7,3+0,1	7,3+0,1	502±16	38,0±04
40-48	9,3+0,2	7,5+0,1	7,5+0,1	521±23	38,6±1,3

Table 3-5 Testicular biometry of zebu bulls

Age/months	Length	Width	Thickness	TVI	SC
12	8,4 ±0,8	3,8±0,6	3,7 ±0,6	115±17	18,2±1,4
24	11,2 ±0,9	5,8±0,2	5,8 ±0,7	360±36	30,0±3,0
36	12,8 ±0,8	6,4±0,5	6,3 ±0,9	519±11	32,0±0,5
48	13,3 ±1,4	8,5±0,6	8,1 ±0,6	926±169	41,0±3,0

Average values ± standard deviation in cm. Age in months.
TVI = testicular volume index. SCR = scrotal circumference.

These results allow the breeder to use testicular size as a selection criterion, since it is expected that a bull with a high VTI or CE may have a higher sperm production than another with lower values.

This is true, but the breeder must interpret the quality of testicular size in its true value, since the most important thing is that the gonads are within the minimum range considered normal for males of the age, build and breed in question.

Experience shows that bulls with larger or more voluminous testicles are not always the best as breeders.

Animal model using the BLUP methodology

The development of the animal model using the BLUP methodology, an acronym for *Best Linear Unbiased Prediction*, is capable of estimating the fixed effects (systematic environmental effects) and predicting the random effects (the genetic values of the candidates for selection).

The BLUP methodology has gradually become popular for evaluating breeding animals based on field data.

Problems with genetic evaluation

Domestic animal populations usually live and reproduce in the same herds throughout their useful life. The livestock practices and their statistical consequences that can most influence the genetic evaluation of animals are:

a) Directed mating

b) Selection

c) Changes in genetic variances

d) The existence of subpopulations with different genetic levels

The most widely used method today is the one known by its acronym BLUP. Although it was originally designed for dairy cattle, it is very frequently used in other species.

The prediction of genetic value is based on the use of information collected in production controls, and the relationship with other animals also included in the control.

With current statistical techniques it is possible to combine all the available information about the production of animals in a population, the environmental circumstances in which these productions took place and the relationships between them, to obtain an estimate of the genetic potential of each individual. The way to combine all this information is through the use of statistical models.

A statistical model is a simplified mathematical description of how the production of an individual takes place based on genetic and environmental considerations.

Linear Models

The correct analysis of a sample of biological data begins with careful reflection and a detailed description of the statistical model.

The BLUP method uses two sources of information to carry out the genetic assessment of an animal, the production data and the genealogy of the animals.

The most notable characteristics of the BLUP methodology would be:

1) **It uses all the available information regarding productions**
   - All the data of the animals are included, both those that are alive and those that are no longer in the herd, but that at some point in the life of the herd had records.

2) It uses all the existing genealogical information

- This information includes the breeding males through their offspring and breeding females that do not have data, but do have offspring with data. In addition to the offspring, information from any other known relative is included.
- Breeding males that have already disappeared, but with offspring in the population, can be used.
- The BLUP methodology uses all the relatives of all the animals in the most efficient way to obtain the genetic value of all the animals included in the database.

The most outstanding properties of the BLUP method are:

1) The BLUP methodology with the animal model takes into account the specific matings that can occur in the different herds

- This is important, as it indicates that the possible directed matings that the breeder may want to make will be taken into account.

2) The genealogy of each animal is a source of information of great importance when it comes to genetically evaluating the animals

- It is evident that, if a stallion has a group of offspring with high weights at a certain age, it is a sign that this male had a different treatment with respect to the other stallions, and this would distort the comparisons between them.

3) **The genetic evaluations obtained through BLUP are referred to a base population whose genetic value is zero**
   - This base population is made up of all those animals with unknown father and mother. If the father and mother of an animal are unknown, the BLUP assumes that it belongs to the base generation and will therefore assign it a different genetic prediction than the one that would correspond to it.

4) **The genetic assessment of an animal will only be useful if it has been obtained with a certain degree of reliability, security or precision**
   - The BLUP provides us with this precision and depends on the amount of information available on each animal. The precision ranges between zero and one.

5) **Changes in genetic variance as a result of selection and inbreeding are taken into account through the genetic variance-covariance matrix**
   - This matrix integrates all the genealogical information, taking into account the pairings and possible inbreeding.

6) **The BLUP methodology for obtaining genetic predictions assumes that the heritability of the trait is known without error**
   - An overestimation of heritability leads to an evaluation based more on production than on genealogy and, on the contrary, an underestimated heritability gives more importance to genealogy. In any case, neither of the two situations leads to optimal evaluations.

Genomic Sciences

Genomics is the set of sciences and techniques dedicated to the comprehensive study of the functioning, content, evolution and origin of genomes.

It is one of the most cutting-edge areas of biology. Genomics uses knowledge derived from different sciences such as molecular biology, biochemistry, computer science, statistics, mathematics, physics, etc.

Genomic sciences have had a significant boom in recent years, especially thanks to advanced DNA sequencing technologies, advances in bioinformatics, and increasingly sophisticated techniques for performing complete genome analyses.

The development of genomics has contributed to the advancement of different fields of science such as medicine, agriculture, etc., thanks to the discovery of gene sequences necessary to produce proteins of medical importance and the comparison of genomic sequences of different organisms.

In several countries such as the United States, the European Union and Japan, enormous projects have been carried out to sequence the genome of various model organisms. Probably the best known is the Human Genome Project.

Today, there are also important public access servers, such as the NCBI (National Center for Biotechnology Information), which allow any user with an Internet connection to access the complete genome sequence of dozens of organisms and the sequences of hundreds of thousands of genes from different organisms.

Unlike classical genetics, which, based on a phenotype (usually a mutant), searches for the gene or genes responsible for said phenotype, genomics aims to predict the function of genes based on their sequence or their interactions with other genes.

Thus, genomics has a different approach to answering biological questions when compared to other, more traditional branches of biology.

Genomic selection

The genome is the totality of the genetic information possessed by a particular organism or species. The genome in eukaryotic beings comprises the DNA contained in the nucleus, organized into chromosomes, and the mitochondrial genome. The term is an acronym for the words gene and chromosome.

Diploid organisms have two copies of the genome in their cells, due to the presence of homologous chromosome pairs. Sex cells are haploid because they only contain one copy.

Sequencing the genome of a species does not analyze the genetic diversity or polymorphism of genes. To study the variations of a gene, comparison between individuals is required through genotyping.

Molecular markers

Molecular analysis techniques that allow the detection of genetic variability directly at the level of the DNA molecule are based on different types of molecular markers.

These genetic markers are used in the construction of genomic maps of different animal species, with a view to detecting and manipulating individual genetic effects of a quantitative nature (quantitative trait loci or QTL) in animal breeding programs, or qualitative effects in studies of disease resistance, racial purity or verification of ancestry.

Livestock farming, and especially that related to the dairy industry, has been a leader in animal production by taking advantage of the fruits of new biotechnological techniques, which will undoubtedly contribute in the coming years to achieving an increase in milk production.

In this industry, the implementation of artificial insemination and embryo transfer have expanded the genetic market, which is joined by the distribution of germplasm from a single parent for the performance of progeny tests in order to study genetic evolution under different management and development conditions.

In animals, we have examples of models developed to evaluate human genetic diseases, the use of animals to produce drugs and as donor sources of cells and organs, for example, the use of animals for the production of human blood proteins or antibodies.

For animal diseases, biotechnology provides numerous opportunities to combat them, and vaccines are being developed against many bovine and porcine diseases, which in recent times have taken their toll on these animals.

This is made possible today, thanks to the new molecular technologies developed, with which the identification of genotypes and the monitoring of animals in populations from markers linked to quantitative traits is achieved.

Genetic polymorphism detection methods

Genetic variability is an attribute that cannot be exhaustively measured. It is impossible to examine each gene in each individual of a given species to obtain a complete enumeration of the species' genetic variation; however, if a sample is taken from a population, it is possible to estimate its genetic variability by using a character or marker that facilitates the measurement of said variability.

Genetic polymorphism or variation of genetic origin has been widely studied in natural populations, as it allows the analysis of phenomena such as the amount of genetic variability and frequency of mutations through characters that are easy to measure and have a known genetic basis, with little influence from the environment on its phenotypic expression.

In determining genetic variability, the "ideal" markers meet a series of characteristics, including high capacity to detect high levels of polymorphism, high heritability, great capacity to access all regions of the genome, independence from the physical and developmental state of the individual, ease of obtaining, detection by economic methods, independence from environmental conditions and the possibility of determination in any type of cell containing a nucleus.

Microsatellite DNA

These are sequences, short DNA fragments that are found very often repeated in certain regions of the genome of eukaryotic cells and whose function is currently unknown. The variations observed in the number of repetitions serve to differentiate two individuals of the same species.

Microsatellites have proven to be the most informative markers for population studies at the subspecies level.

Most of the studies carried out to date with this type of markers are based on the analysis of allelic frequencies, with the aim initially of creating genetic maps and later for determining QTLs.

What is a QTL?

QTL stands for ***Quantitative Trait Loci***, which designates the region of the chromosome that influences a quantitative trait.

A region is sought that contains a gene that has an important effect on a quantitative trait. This means that this gene presents a polymorphism; each form of this gene produces different effects.

Markers are used when the gene has not been directly identified. 3 to 5 QTL per trait of interest. These are large regions that have between 30 and 500 genes.

Examples of QTL to select qualitative traits are shown in the following tables:

Table 3-6 QTLs for cattle

	Cattle	
QTL	**Name**	**Characteristics**
CAPN1	μ-Calpain	Beef tenderness
CAST	Calpastatin	Beef tenderness
LEP	Leptin	Carcass fattening
TG	Thyroglobulin	Intramuscular fattening
DGAT1	Diacylglycerol acetyltransferase	Milk composition
MSTN	Myostatin	Double musculature
IFNG	Interferon gamma	Nematode resistance
GHR	Growth hormone receptor	Weaning and carcass weight

Table 3-7 QTLs for sheep

	Sheep	
QTL	**Name**	**Characteristics**
PRNP	Scrapie prion protein	Resistance/susceptibility
BOF	Callipyge gene	Muscle/meat production
FecX	Inverdale	Fertility in Romey
FecB	Booroola gene	Prolificacy in Merino
FGFR3	Spider leg syndrome	Skeletal abnormality
IFNG	Without Interferon gamma	Resistance to nematodes

Uses:

1. Disease resistance
2. Carcass quality and palatability attributes
3. Fertility and reproductive efficiency
4. Carcass quantity and carcass yield
5. Milk production and maternal ability
6. Growth performance

Because of the importance that these markers have taken in the development of genetic maps, the methods of detection are very variable and new techniques are constantly appearing. Mini satellites are associated with structural characteristics of chromosomes.

A *DNA chip* is a solid surface to which a collection of DNA fragments is attached. The surfaces used to fix the DNA are very variable and can be made of glass, plastic and even silicon.

DNA chips are used to analyze the differential expression of genes, monitoring the levels of thousands of them simultaneously.

Its operation basically consists of measuring the level of hybridization between the specific probe and the target molecule, generally indicated by fluorescence and analyzed by image analysis, which will indicate the level of expression of the gene.

They are usually used to identify genes with differential expression under different conditions. For example, to detect genes that produce certain diseases by comparing the levels of expression between healthy cells and cells that are developing certain types of diseases.

Some applications of molecular markers in livestock farming

This biotechnology is being used in various fields of animal production and health.

Among its main applications in livestock farming are the identification and checking of kinship, the construction of genetic maps, the development of new treatments for diseases.

Molecular markers today constitute a modern and powerful tool for the old art of selection. Among its most immediate applications are the identification of kinship or identity and the characterization of genetic diversity.

In countries with a high level of livestock development and especially in species of economic interest, specifically cattle and horses, genetic identification and the mandatory establishment of paternity tests are beyond any doubt as an argument for the reliability and credibility of the genealogical books for the different breeds.

The importance of animal diseases as the main obstacle to increasing livestock productivity will grow considerably, as animal production intensifies, and livestock density increases in warmer and more humid ecological zones.

The application of DNA biotechnology to animal health, through more effective, cheaper and more resistant vaccines combined with better diagnostic instruments, could contribute significantly to improving disease control, thus stimulating national food production and participation in livestock trade.

Biotechnology also offers considerable possibilities for improving the production of agro-industrial products, especially through environmentally friendly and energy efficient processes.

Although most of these technologies will probably not be within the reach of traditional livestock production, they will be considerably accessible to the emerging commercial and industrial sector in developing countries.

Predictive value of genomic selection

Genomic selection allows the genetic value of the animal to be predicted from the moment of birth with a degree of reliability of around 70 %, since it combines genomic predictions with genotypes, phenotypes and pedigree data.

This selection constitutes a tool that has generated enormous interest and expectations in the field of genetic improvement worldwide and, above all, in dairy cattle, where it has been used with greater emphasis until now.

In addition, with GEBV, the reliability of the tests is increased, the generation interval is reduced, and the intensity of the selection is increased (Table 3-6 and 3-7).

Genomic selection significantly improves the reliability of the genetic values of the bulls in test and especially those with few descendants; This increase in reliability will provide great advantages when selecting the parents of bulls and cows, thus causing an increase in genetic progress.

Genomic selection does not completely replace performance and genealogy controls, so it is essential to collect and have the phenotypes and productive data of the selected animals.

The genetic value of the individuals obtained by GEBV offers some advantages compared to the indices generated by traditional genetic evaluations.

These are:

1. The genetic potential of an animal can be known early on, which only requires taking a biological sample that is easy to obtain (hair, blood).

2. It allows everyone to be studied at a genomic level, helping to discriminate between full siblings who, because both parents are the same, tend to reflect very similar genetic indices, even without having to perform progeny tests.

3. It provides greater reliability compared to traditional genetic evaluations, especially in traits with low heritability. In this way, there is a lower risk that the animal's progeny test will show a genetic value very different from that which it had at birth.

4. The use of high-density chips can provide better estimates of homozygosity and therefore avoid close inbreeding, and generate genetically more diverse breeding animals than those selected based only on phenotypes such as those generated through BLUP

Chapter 4

Mating Systems

Contents:
Introduction. Random mating. Mating according to phenotypic similarity. Mating according to the genetic relationship between individuals. Crossbreeding or outbreeding. Genetic and phenotypic effects of crossing.

Introduction

It is known that the genetic structure of populations is determined by gene and genotypic frequencies and that the factors that produce changes in the latter are migration, mutation, selection and genetic drift. Another factor that influences genotypic frequency is the mating system applied in the population. This system by itself does not alter gene frequencies because it does not involve parental selection. If females and males' mate without considering genetic or phenotypic similarity, then mating is random, and the genotypic frequencies of the offspring will remain in Hardy-Weinberg equilibrium. When mating considers the phenotypic similarity to the genetic relationships between individuals, a direct effect on the genetic structure of the population occurs and the frequencies of the different genotypes deviate from the population in genetic equilibrium. Each of the systems produces a particular effect on the genetic structure of the population, which will be analyzed below.

Random mating

Each male in the population has an equal opportunity to mate with each female and vice versa. The consequence of this type of mating is offspring in Hardy-Weinberg genetic equilibrium. This type of natural mating is the one carried out by animals in the wild and in extensive breeding of domestic ruminant herds.

Mating according to phenotypic similarity

It occurs in two ways: when the individuals that mate are very similar, or they are very different phenotypically.

In the first case, the mated animals have greater phenotypic similarity than if they had been randomly selected from the population to which they belong, for example, if in a herd AA coat males are mated with AA females, SS males with BS coat females and AB males with AS females.

This mating leads to changes in the genotypic frequency of the offspring. That is, in the first generation the frequency of the AS heterozygote is reduced by half compared to the base population and the AA and SS homozygotes increase by 25 %.

The genetic effect of this type of mating on qualitative traits is to change the genotypic frequency, producing an increase in the frequency of homozygotes (AA) and (BB), and a decrease in heterozygotes (AB).

In quantitative traits, only slight changes occur on the genotypic frequency and the main effect is the increase in the genetic variability of the trait. In addition, it reduces the rate at which the population reaches the equilibrium for linkage.

Mating between different individuals is the opposite of the previous one, that is, animals are mated that are less similar than if they had been chosen at random in the population to which they belong. Its genetic effect is also the opposite, increasing the frequency of heterozygous genotypes and decreasing that of homozygotes. In this case, the population can reach a state of equilibrium in which all genotypes are represented, but less frequently for homozygotes.

If in practice one were to try to make the population of cattle more uniform, for example, by mating small cows with large bulls and *vice versa*, one is applying mating between less similar individuals.

Mating according to the genetic relationship between individuals

Inbreeding and outcrossing are the mating systems that are based mainly on the degree of genetic relationship that exists between individuals.

Inbreeding

This is the mating of animals that are more closely related than the average of the population to which they belong. Inbreeding is said to exist when the individuals that mate are genetically related (related).

However, expressed in this way, the concept may not be precisely defined. For example, if parents and children, siblings, or grandparents and grandchildren are mated, it would be clear that these are consanguineous pairings, although with different degrees. When the mating occurs between parents and children or between siblings, it is said that the consanguinity is close.

If the sexual union occurs between half-siblings, uncles, cousins, or other distant relatives, it is said that the consanguinity is collateral. In these cases, these genetic relationships between individuals are not so evident.

In a population, all the individuals that mate could be genetically related, at least in a slight or remote way. The genetic relationships of the individuals that make up the population will depend on the size of the population.

In a bisexual population, everyone has two parents, four grandparents, eight great-grandparents, and so on, doubling the number of ancestors in each generation, and *t* generations back it will have **2t** ancestors.

Thus, for example, in 10 generations (210) an animal will have more than a thousand ancestors in its pedigree if there is no inbreeding. If two animals are not related, then in the last 10 generations they would logically each have to have more than a thousand different ancestors.

This means that any pair of individuals could therefore be related to each other, through one or more common ancestors, in a more or less remote past.

Logically, the smaller the population size in previous generations, the less remote the common ancestors will be or the greater their number. Randomly mated pairs are more closely related to each other in a small population than in a large population.

Inbreeding coefficient

A measure of inbreeding is the *inbreeding coefficient*. This has been defined in various ways and takes values from zero to one.

F is definable as: "The correlation between the genetic values of the gametes that unite", or as: "the probability that two genes at the same locus are identical by descent."

Recalling the concepts of gene identity, this definition is equivalent to "the probability that two alleles of a locus entering the zygote will come from a common ancestral allele."

At a particular locus, genes may or may not be identical by descent. However, considering all loci, **F** expresses what proportion of these loci carry identical genes by descent. **F** can also be defined as the proportion of loci that were heterozygous in the base population and have become homozygous.

Calculation of the coefficient of inbreeding (F)

The following exemplifies the calculation of the coefficient of inbreeding (**F**) from the pedigree illustrated.

The coefficient of inbreeding of individual **X** is 0.160, which expressed as a percentage would be 16 %. According to the definitions of F_1, this means that the probability that **X** has a pair of genes identical by descent at a locus is 16 %; or also, that 16 % of the loci that were heterozygous in the base population have become homozygous.

The base population is the one taken as the starting point for the calculation. It may be made up of the animals in which the experiment was started or with which a herd or a certain breed was founded, or it may be made up of individuals born on a certain date. When an individual belongs to the base population, it is assumed that it has a consanguinity equal to zero.

When the consanguinity coefficient is calculated in the manner described above, the base population to which it refers must be defined, otherwise said coefficient would lack its true value.

Example:

A population is considered in Hardy-Weinberg equilibrium with gene frequencies: $A_1=0.4$ and $A_2=0.6$; and genotypic frequencies: $A_1A_1=0.16$; $A_1A_2=0.48$; $A_2A_2=0.36$. If the genealogy of this population is not known, it can be assumed that all its members have an **F**=0. In this population the probability that an individual is homozygous is: 0.16+0.36=0.52; but they are considered to be genes equal in state, rather than identical by descent, that is, independent homozygotes.

If an individual **X** has an inbreeding coefficient of F_x=0.3, relative to this base population, then the probability that he is heterozygous at a locus is 1-0.3=0.7 of the probability that a randomly selected member of the base population is heterozygous, that is, 0.7x0.48=0.34.

If in this example the inbreeding of **X** were zero, then **X** would have a probability of 0.48 of being heterozygous, that is, the same as the base population.

An alternative to determine the exponents of ½ in the formula is to count individuals instead of generations. Thus, **n** will be equal to the number of individuals, starting with the link initiated with individual **L**, passing through the parent **d** to the common ancestor **A** and so on. This one towards the other parent **e** and y towards **b**.

The coefficients will be written: $F_x = \sum (½)^n (1 + F_A)$

When it comes to **F**, the count begins with the parents.

Inbreeding systems

The effects of inbreeding are similar to those of mating between phenotypically similar individuals, since both tend to increase homozygosity and decrease heterozygosity.

The fundamental difference lies in that inbreeding increases homozygosity in all segregating genes and in the other case the genotypic frequencies change only for the loci that cause the variation in the trait on which the mating is based according to phenotypic similarity (and for the genes linked to said loci).

As a consequence of the increase in homozygosity, the frequency of all defects and abnormalities, determined by recessive genes, increases.

Most defects and abnormalities decrease the productive and reproductive performance of animals. The fundamental effects resulting from the increase in homozygosity are:

a) **Fixation of traits.** When absorbing crosses are performed, it is observed that in the fifth generation 48.4 % of the population is homozygous A_1A_1. The mating within these individuals, together with the inbreeding process, will tend to fix the A_1 allele within this subgroup of individuals. The same will happen with the other segregating allele A_2.

b) **Formation of lines.** As a result of inbreeding, the population is divided into subgroups or lines. All the lines come from the base population and in each of them the alleles that pass to the homozygous state are different. Therefore, as inbreeding continues to apply, the genetic differences between lines are greater and the genetic variance within the lines decreases. The total additive genetic variance (V_A) increases. This is because there are greater differences between homozygous individuals for different genes (A_1A_1 vs. A_2A_2) than between individuals carrying these genes in heterozygosity (A_1A_2).

c) **The initial frequency** of rare genes increases in some lines. The total genetic variance due to rare genes increases linearly with **F**.

In addition to the changes described for genetic variance, changes in phenotypic variance occur in inbred populations. It has been found that, in highly inbred lines, individuals are very variable in their phenotypic values for some quantitative traits, such as, for example, size and weight at a certain age; it has also been observed that individuals from crosses between lines tend to be more uniform in their phenotypic values.

If animals within an inbred line are generally more similar, these differences can be attributed to environmental causes.

Inbred animals are generally less resistant to adverse environmental effects, which can lead to an increase in environmental variance.

It is estimated that inbred animals have a lower capacity to adjust their developmental and physiological mechanisms to various environmental changes. This is evidenced by greater loss in early life stages, lower reproductive capacity, and a slower growth rate.

Uses of inbreeding

The most limiting factor for the use of inbreeding in animal breeding is the decrease in vigor that accompanies it. However, there are certain circumstances in which it can be applied:

- 1- To check whether the breeders that have been evaluated based on their productive traits are carriers or not of deleterious (lethal) genes.

2- To select against a recessive gene of economic importance. Since inbreeding reveals hidden recessive genes, homozygous recessive and heterozygous individuals can be identified and eliminated.

3- To develop lines within a breed, for later crossing with a view to exploiting the heterosis produced. This is currently the main use of inbreeding.

4- To fix characters in the process of forming new breeds.

Inbreeding depression

When inbreeding is too close and is maintained over several generations, a depressing effect on the performance of most traits may occur and cause deterioration in the general vigor and health of the animals. The effect of lethal genes and undesirable traits also appear more frequently.

The origin of inbreeding depression can be derived from the expression given for the population mean:

$$Mp = a(p - q) + 2pqd$$

Inbreeding decreases the proportion of heterozygotes, so the mean of the population with an inbreeding coefficient F will be:

$$M_F = a(p - q) + 2pqd(1 - F)$$
$$M_F = Mp - 2pqdF$$

The reduction in the mean phenotypic value of traits related to reproductive capacity or physiological efficiency is called inbreeding depression.

Not all traits show inbreeding depression to the same degree. Those related to reproductive rate or fitness show greater sensitivity, for example, litter size in pigs, egg number and hatchability in chickens, and fertility in cattle. These traits generally have low inheritance rates and show a high degree of heterosis when crossbreeding occurs.

In other traits, such as milk fat content, egg size in chickens, there is little or no change. Growth rate shows a greater decrease than the above. These traits have medium to high inheritance rates and show low heterosis when crossbreeding.

In dairy cattle, for example, it has been shown that there is generally a depressive effect on milk and fat production, growth and reproductive performance. A decrease of approximately 22.5 kg of milk has been observed for each increase in **F**=0.01. Losses of this magnitude are high, and even considering that there are no other effects, it is clear that the use of inbred bulls is not advisable.

Inbreeding reduces birth weight by about 0.11 kg for each increase in **F**=0.01. In addition, in inbred populations, more services are required per conception and puberty is delayed, thus decreasing multiple ovulations.

In dairy cattle, father-son mating and other close inbreeding systems increase female mortality by almost 50 %.

The depressive effects described are a limitation for the application of inbreeding. However, some degree of inbreeding is required when it comes to traits to which selection must be applied for improvement.

In dairy cattle, to avoid mating between related individuals, the intensity of selection will decrease. Therefore, the best breeding bulls, that is, those with the greatest genetic superiority, should be used, but considering their relationship with the population.

The effects of inbreeding on fertility, viability, sexual maturity, pre-weaning growth and maternal ability are also evident in beef cattle.

Crossbreeding or outbreeding

In practice, it refers to the mating between individuals that have not had common ancestors in four or five generations prior to their birth.

It is also defined as the mating between two individuals that are less closely related to each other than the average of the population to which they belong.

The concept includes mating between individuals that come from different lines within the same breed; or from different breeds and when reproductive continuity between species allows it.

Through crossbreeding, several favorable effects are obtained, which together increase the efficiency of animal production. Among the main advantages are:

a) **Presence of heterosis or hybrid vigor**, a phenomenon resulting from the combination of two or more genotypes in a certain cross, in which the phenotypic value of the offspring can exceed the average of the populations that gave rise to it and is sometimes higher than the average of the best parent. In Zoogenetics it is more appropriate to use the term heterosis since the hybrid is the offspring of the coupling between species.

b) **Complementarity.** A favorable result of the average effect of the genotypes that were combined in the cross to maximize the merit of the offspring, in its total productivity.

c) **Greater resistance** to some diseases and particular environmental conditions.

Species, races, strains and families

The basic units in animal systematics are the species that are represented by groups of animals which have specific characteristics in the structure of the body, which are common to all animals within each group where they mate and reproduce with each other.

The differences between species are fundamentally marked by reproductive discontinuity, that is, if individuals of different species mate, they will not reproduce; otherwise, the offspring will be infertile.

However, this reproductive continuity has different degrees of manifestation, with various mechanisms acting, some occurring before fertilization occurs and others after mating.

Examples of these mechanisms are, among others: isolation in the habitat, the impossibility of fertilization due to incompatibility in the genitals, genetic mortality or non-viability of the hybrid and the sterility of the crossed offspring.

As already stated, in Zoogenetics the individuals resulting from the mating between species are called *hybrids*. The result of the mating between the horse and the donkey species are the hybrids called *mule* and *hinny*; the former being widely used commercially as a pack animal.

In this coupling, the mare's eggs are fertilized by the donkey's sperm and from these fertilization mules are born. The male offspring are sterile and some fertile females have been produced exceptionally.

From the coupling between the donkey and the horse the hinny is born, which does not have the qualities of size and resistance of the mule.

Sheep and goats present wider genetic differences than in the previous case and when animals of these two species are mated, the fertilization of the egg occurs, but the embryo does not develop completely and is reabsorbed.

On the other hand, there are groups of animals that differ widely in the average value of many of their traits and yet, when mated, reproduce without difficulty. This is the case of Bos taurus and Bos indicus, with both the female and male offspring being fertile. These groups, which are related by intermediate individuals (which are produced when they are crossed), are defined as subspecies of the same species and therefore their offspring are crossbred and not hybrids.

Species are subdivided into races. A race can be defined as a population that is different from others by its gene and genotypic frequencies.

The description of a race implies complete information about all its genes and genotypes, or at least about the most important ones.

Such a description of a race is practically impossible and therefore the specification is always a description of the morphological traits that characterize it, such as biotype, color, type of hair, etc., which are of high h^2 independent of the environment. However, most breeds differ in traits that are of economic importance, such as milk production, milk fat percentage, meat production, etc., which are highly influenced by the environment, which increases their variances and causes overlapping in the distribution of various breeds.

The quantitative traits of a breed can be characterized by their averages and not by their individual values.

Since quantitative traits depend on a large number of genes and, therefore, there is a considerable degree of heterozygosity within each breed, biologically there are no "pure breeds" and it is practically impossible to achieve them.

Pure breed

This is the term used for animals that, fulfilling the established racial pattern, are registered in the genealogical books.

Not all animals of a species can be included in a specific breed and in addition to the so-called pure breeds, there are others that come from the crossing of two breeds called *crossbreds* or *mestizos*.

Breeds are divided into subpopulations called *strains*, which refers to the set of animals within a breed that have been selected for a specific purpose and are kept away from other groups that belong to the same breed.

Line

A group of animals that have a higher degree of homozygosity, because of consanguineous mating.

If a line reaches a coefficient of consanguinity of at least 0.375, which corresponds to the mating between siblings for two generations, it is called a *consanguineous line*.

Family

A *family* is understood as the set of ancestors, descendants, collaterals and relatives of a lineage.

Genetic and phenotypic effects of crossing

The main effect of crossing on the genetic structure of populations is the change in the genotypic frequencies of the crossed generation, producing an increase in the proportion of heterozygous genotypes at the expense of the decrease of homozygotes.

Heterosis

The deviation of the average phenotypic value shown by the crossed progeny (in one or more characters) compared to the average phenotypic value of the parental populations or of one of them is called *heterosis* or also *hybrid vigor*.

It is observed that when two inbred lines are crossed, the offspring show an increase in the phenotypic value of those traits that previously suffered from "*inbreeding depression*". Likewise, it has been shown that the loss of the "*selective value*" or "*adaptive value*", which occurs because of inbreeding, tends to be recovered through crossbreeding.

The effect of heterosis depends on the changes in genotypic frequency, described above, and can manifest itself as a result of the mating of inbred lines within a breed, as well as by the crossing between different breeds. However, some differences must be taken into account in this regard.

When measuring heterosis from the crossing between inbred lines, the value obtained are more notable, which is since the offspring are compared with inbred parents that have a lower performance for the traits affected by inbreeding depression.

In crosses between breeds, heterosis represents an improvement in the performance of the progeny, which is superior to the average of pure commercial herds; or also superior to the best of them.

Genetic diversity between breeds is also more favored (than between lines within breeds) to produce suitable genetic combinations, given the variations in the production-management complex, since each breed has been subject to a long process of natural and artificial selection that has provided it with some specialized adaptation.

On the other hand, the development of inbred lines produces additional costs that must be equated with the greater effectiveness of the crossbred progeny, to justify their use.

Heterosis in the F_1

The amount of heterosis is expressed as the difference between the average of the F_1 and the parental average, that is:

$$H_F = M_F - M_p$$
$$H_F = d y^2$$

If it is assumed that the genotypic values attributed to each locus combine additively, the heterosis produced y the sum of each particular contribution can be represented.

Thus, the heterosis in the F_1 would be:

$$H_{F_1} = \sum d\, y^2$$

The following conclusions can be drawn from this expression:

A. The amount of heterosis that occurs in the F_1 progeny depends on the type of gene action that acts on the segregating loci and on the difference in gene frequency of the populations involved in the crossing.

This means that the greater the difference in gene frequency of the populations that are crossed, the greater the degree of heterosis shown for a given value of *d*. The greatest effect should be expected when each allele is fixed in a different population.

For heterosis to occur, the value of *d* must be different from zero, therefore, if the additivity of the genes predominates, the manifestation of this effect should not be expected.

On the other hand, directional dominance must be considered, that is, if several loci are dominant in one direction and others in the opposite direction, heterosis will not be manifested. Therefore, if a character does not show heterosis, it cannot be concluded that it does not present dominance in the loci individually.

It should be expected that traits determined by loci in which gene action is dominance or over-dominance will show more heterosis than those in which the additive effect of the genes predominates.

If an allele determining the increase of a quantitative trait has a value greater than zero for d (partially or totally dominant or over-dominant), then the effect of the crossing is to increase the population mean. But when d takes a negative value, the mean in the crossed progeny may be lower than the average of the parental populations.

Heterosis in the F_2

The random mating of the individuals of the F_1 will produce an F_2 progeny in Hardy-Weinberg equilibrium, where the genotypic frequency will be determined by the gene frequency in the F_1.

The mean in F_2 is obtained by applying the following formula:

$$M_{F_2} = a\,(p - \tfrac{1}{2}y - q - \tfrac{1}{2}y) + 2\,d\,(p - \tfrac{1}{2}y)(q + \tfrac{1}{2}y)$$
$$M_{F_2} = a\,(p - q - y) + d\,[\,2pq + y(p - q) - \tfrac{1}{2}y^2\,]$$

The amount of heterosis shown by the F_2 will be given by the difference between the mean of the F_2 and the mean of the parental populations.

$$H_{F2} = M_{F2} - M_p = \tfrac{1}{2} d\, y^2$$
$$H_{F2} = \tfrac{1}{2} F_1$$

That is, theoretically, the amount of heterosis shown in the F_2 generation is reduced by half compared to that obtained in the F_1 generation.

The analysis carried out considering a character determined by a single locus allows to define the possible genetic causes that determine heterosis, namely, non-additive effect of the genes and difference in gene frequency between populations.

However, most of the characteristics of economic interest such as: milk, meat or egg production; fertility, prolificacy and others, are quantitative and are influenced by genes in many loci and the number of genes or the frequency in which they are found is unknown.

It is likely that in these traits non-additive gene interactions, such as epistasis, also contribute to heterosis. For this reason, it should not be absolutely assumed that the total heterosis presented by a quantitative trait is due only to the sum of the heterotic effects produced by the segregating loci and to the differences in gene frequencies shown by the populations for the trait in question. $\sum d\, y^2$

Types of heterosis

Individual heterosis

This is the amount of hybrid vigor attributable to the heterozygosity of the crossbred progeny and which is measurable in the progeny itself.

When crossbreeding occurs, the parental populations are not always purebreds, and in many cases crossbred mothers are used.

The advantage or heterosis obtained in the progeny, due to the heterozygosity of the crossbred mothers, is called *maternal heterosis*.

If, for example, crossbred sheep have better maternal ability than purebred sheep, this effect could be reflected in a higher survival rate, or higher pre-weaning growth rate, in the lambs. It is also possible that in crossbred cows (for meat production), individual heterosis occurs for milk production, which would be reflected as maternal heterosis in the pre-weaning growth of the calves.

Paternal heterosis

This is the additional effect that occurs in the offspring when crossbred parents are used, compared to purebred parents.

It is possible to specify that there are three types of heterosis: *individual*, *maternal* and *paternal*, which can be combined to produce a greater effect on the phenotypic value of the crossbred offspring.

Maternal effects

Maternal influences are an important source of variation in mammals. The maternal effect has a double origin; it is environmental in relation to the offspring, but it depends on the mother's genotype and its association with the effects of the environment.

The maternal environmental effect that females exert on their offspring can be differentiated in two stages: prenatal and postnatal.

Prenatal stage. Period from ovulation to birth

The mother can influence the traits of her offspring at birth, by the uterine environment that she provides to her fetus, as well as by the genes that she transmits to it.

This effect, which is attributable to variations in the uterine environment, is not measured directly in the population, but through experimental evaluations, such as the comparison of reciprocal crosses and others.

Examples of traits affected by the uterine environment: litter size and birth weight of the offspring.

Postnatal effects. Period from birth to weaning

In mammalian offspring, the pre-weaning growth rate depends largely on the milk production of the mothers.

In beef cattle, for example, this effect can accelerate or delay the pre-weaning growth of calves and therefore one of the traits to be evaluated in cows is *maternal ability*.

The maternal effect is one of the factors that contribute to the value of heterosis. In the previous example, the greater milk production of the crossbred mother could increase the effect of heterosis and vice versa.

In experiments carried out on crosses of Zebu breeds with European breeds for beef production, crossbred cows with excellent maternal aptitude are produced. They are good dairy producers, with high fertility and wean a greater proportion of their own weight in the form of calves than pure tropical or European breeds.

The differences between breeds due to the maternal effect become an advantage when the appropriate cross is chosen. These differences are the basis of complementarity. There is a lot of evidence showing the existence of heterosis when crossbreeding occurs in different species.

In many crossbreeds, maternal lines that have been specialized for maternal traits and paternal lines specialized for the characteristics of interest in animals for slaughter are used.

The effects of *complementarity* vary depending on the differences shown by the paternal populations in productive and reproductive behavior, as well as the direction in which the crossing is carried out.

The genetic gains obtained through crossing are given by the joint effects of heterosis and complementarity between races.

Crossing systems

Below, the crosses that are most used in different species will be described and analyzed.

Each system has its particularities and to choose which cross to carry out, the genetic aspects will be taken into consideration, as well as the general characteristics of the production system under which the crossed animals will be raised.

When describing crosses, reference is made to the broader concept of the population, taking into account that it can be: lines or varieties within a race; different races or populations that are a mixture of different races.

The *population* can be defined as a group of individuals that mate with each other and have in common a set of genes that characterize and differentiate it from other groups.

Discontinuous or specific crosses

Cross between two populations

The A and B races are crossed and the F_1 (AB) progeny is produced. The F_1 progeny resulting from the cross must show the highest degree of heterozygosity, since on average it has one gene of type A and another of type B at any loci, which favors the best expression of hybrid vigor or individual heterosis.

This type of cross does not take advantage of the benefits of maternal heterosis, since none of the parental populations is crossed.

The average phenotypic value in the offspring of the F_1 cross is determined by the average of the genes contributed by each parent, the average of the genes that determine the maternal effect in the maternal race, and by the individual heterosis shown by said progeny. In the absence of the heterosis effect, the phenotypic value of the F_1 (AS) will be intermediate between the paternal races. The objective of this cross is to obtain a high level of efficiency in commercial production based on hybrid vigor.

Its application is limited when the reproductive rate of the species is low, as, for example, in cattle, since then it is necessary to maintain the breeding of the herds of the parental breeds, to guarantee the continuity of the crossbreeding and the replacement of the crossed progeny.

Also generally the crossing of two breeds is applied as a starting point for schemes of greater complexity; in Cuba, in cattle, the crossing of Zebu cows with Holstein bulls was used to produce the F_1 (H x C) from which a broad crossing program was developed to obtain new breeds.

The differences between reciprocal crossbreeds have three probable causes:

a) The existence of extra-chromosomal DNA
b) The genes linked to sex

c) The maternal effect of an environmental type that occurs on progeny

The latter is the most interesting from a practical point of view.

This cross can also provide the advantages of *complementarity*, which is maximized when female and male parents are used, which always come respectively from the same population. When this happens, the parental populations are called *maternal line* and *paternal line*.

The terms maternal line and paternal line are used to indicate the contribution of each breed or genotype to the cross in question.

Backcross

It refers to the mating of F_1 (AB) cross progeny with one of the parental breeds.

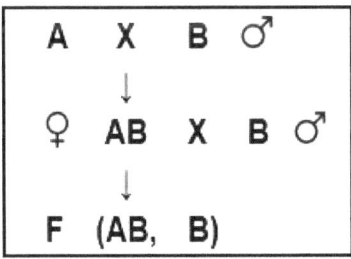

Crossed females are mainly used for backcrossing, in order to take advantage of the effect of maternal heterosis that they show and that favors the traits related to fertility and maternal ability.

The crossed female is 100 % heterozygous, since it has an A gene and a B gene in any locus, and the maximum possible heterosis will be produced. Likewise, the progeny of the F (AB, B) backcross is the result of the union of a B gamete that contains all the B genes and another AB gamete that contains an A gene and a B gene. Therefore, the offspring of the backcross have on average, two BB genes in half of their loci, that is, they are homozygous; and the other half of their loci, one A gene and one B gene, that is, they are heterozygous.

In this way, the backcross is, on average, 50 % less heterozygous and, therefore, the heterosis that it shows can be reduced by 50 %.

Crossing three populations

F_1 (AB) crossed females are mated with males of a third C race.

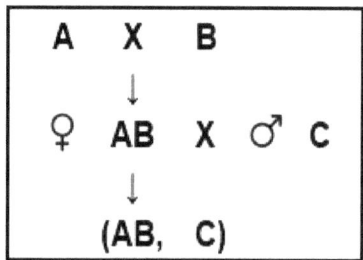

The use of heterosis and complementarity between breeds is maximized. The heterosis of the F crossbred females (AB) used as mothers and favoring traits related to fertility and maternal ability are combined with the individual heterosis of the F crossbred progeny (ABC).

Breeds A and B can be chosen for their maternal trait merits and would be mated to males of breed E, chosen for individual traits such as growth rate, feed efficiency and carcass quality.

Three-breed crossbreeding is used extensively in the poultry industry and is also applied in pig breeding.

Continuous crossbreeding

Rotational

Crossbred females are mated to males of either of the parent breeds or others, alternating matings in each new generation. Two, three, four or more breeds may be included.

Absorption Cross

Before we get into this section, it is convenient to clarify some concepts that can lead to confusion.

It is a widespread custom among breeders, and even among many technicians, to say that individuals from the first generation have half-blood of the improved breed or that they are half-blood; that those from the second generation have three-quarters of improved blood; those from the third, seven-eighths, and so on, as if the quality of the blood of each individual from a given generation were the result of an arithmetic operation.

This concept is erroneous, even in the figurative sense, interpreting the word blood not in its real meaning of blood tissue, but in a broader sense, as representative of the nature of the individual in general.

This nature, made up of the set of qualitative and quantitative characteristics of the individual, depends on the genotype to which it belongs and we already know how variable this can be with the same number of parents: this variability means that an individual can in some cases possess characteristics exactly intermediate between those of its parents and in many others be further away or closer to one of them than to the other.

This idea is equally applicable to absorbent crossing as to any other type of crossing, but we have stopped at it here because the qualification of the descendant, by the supposed fraction of the improving race that is possessed, is more frequently applied when this type of cross is made.

The use of this fractional nomenclature, as widespread as it is erroneous, would only be admissible in a conventional way as an indicator of the intervention of the parents of the improved race in the previous generations of a given individual, but in no case as representative of the quality of the individual in question. This, in fact, cannot be divided into halves, quarters, or eighths, according to its qualities or even its productive possibilities.

The number of generations cannot serve as a criterion to determine the proportion in which the genes of the improved breed appear in the genotype of the descendant, since the composition of this genotype depends on the genetic contribution of the gametes to the zygote, and this can also be extremely varied.

Despite this clarification, we will continue to use this nomenclature in a conventional way, so as not to break with the patterns established by practice.

Absorption crossing

Successive backcrosses are carried out from one population to another, with the objective of introducing new genes into the population with the purpose of replacing one population with another.

In Cuba, this method was applied to obtain the so-called tropical Holstein and the Cuban Charolais. These new breeds still maintain a small percentage of zebu genes in their genotype.

This system is quite efficient in the use of the reproductive capacity of the breed that is being replaced and also has the economic advantage that only stallions or semen of the exotic breed are required to replace the local cattle.

In general, crosses in the first generation (F_1) present the highest yields. It has been observed that the second generation of absorption yields less than the proportions of ½ or ⅝ of the introduced breed, decreasing the "hybrid vigor" when proportions higher than ¾ or ⅞ of the exotic breeds are reached.

In the analysis of other traits such as mortality of crossbred cows, percentage of abortions and percentage of cows culled before calving, the superiority of the cross with 50 % Holstein is evident.

Synthetic populations

This is another alternative for the use of differences between breeds. It is defined as a population mixed from two or more populations, with the same or different proportion of genes from the parental populations.

These populations can be specialized for certain traits and then used as a maternal line or paternal line, thus taking advantage of the effects of complementarity; or they can be used in a general way.

The parent breeds or populations that will give rise to synthetic populations must be previously evaluated for traits of economic importance and for specific environments (climate, nutrition, production systems), as well as for their combining abilities in order to obtain the optimal proportion of genes and the greatest production and adaptation of subsequent crossed generations.

There are two general methods of forming these populations: open or closed.

Open synthetic populations

"*Native*" populations receive genes from "*superior animals*" belonging to exotic populations.

It is an immigration of individuals or entire populations (using artificial insemination or embryo transfer techniques, this work is facilitated). A crossbred population is then formed within which selection is carried out.

In the pig species, this type of open synthetic populations has been developed, with the number of breeds involved in its formation being variable. Thus, for example, at the Experimental Animal Breeding Station in Edinburgh, a synthetic paternal line was created by applying immigration combined with selection.

For eleven generations, immigrants of any of the breeds involved in the program were mated to pigs from the paternal line, regardless of breed, and their offspring were given the same chance of being selected as the offspring of native breeds.

After the eleventh generation, the paternal line consisted of:

- Large White (30%); British Landrace (22%); Norwegian Landrace (20%); Pietrian (10%); American Yorkshire (7%); Hampshire (4%); Tamworth (2%); Wesser Saddleback (2%); Lacombe (2%); commercial crossbreds (1%).

This paternal line showed advantages in the traits: growth rate, feed efficiency, lean meat percentage; compared to the contemporary Large White breed. Back fat was similar to pure breeds and there were no differences in reproductive performance.

Closed synthetic populations

The parents are crossed to obtain a mixed population that has the optimal proportions. The population is then closed and selection begins within it. The effectiveness of this result will depend on the behavior and combining ability of the genotypes that were chosen.

In general, once the synthetic population has been formed, the objective is to improve it by carrying out selection within it as quickly as possible.

The result of selection within a synthetic population may be the creation of a new breed; for example, in cattle, the Santa Gertrudis, Siboney de Cuba, etc. breeds are breeds formed from selection within synthetic populations.

In these cases, it is very important to keep the effective size of the population large enough to avoid the appearance of inbreeding and its adverse effects, which would cancel out the advantages of heterozygosity that initially occurred with the crossing.

New breed crossing

The formation of new breeds is another way to take advantage of genetic differences between breeds.

The objective of new breeds is to achieve optimal combinations of desired characteristics that the parental populations separately present and that also adapt better to environmental conditions.

In this cross, additive genetic effects are used and part of the heterosis that occurs in the F_1 generation is retained, from which the different programs are developed.

Most of the breeds recognized today come from the crossing of two or more breeds or populations and there are numerous examples in the different species.

The new breeds generally have certain advantages, although this does not mean that they are the solution to all needs. The Santa Gertrudis, for example, has a good growth rate and rusticity, but some males have a defective libido and long intervals between births occur in the females.

Also in the Jamaica Hope there are limitations in reproductive efficiency, which seems to be related to the inbreeding applied at its foundation.

The consolidation of a new breed requires a certain degree of inbreeding with intensive selection after the crosses carried out for its fertilization and, in addition, *inter se* crosses, for three or four generations. That is, mating males of the same new breed with newly established females.

Example:

The offspring of a ⅝ Holstein x ⅜ Zebu heifer must be mated with a purebred bull of the Siboney de Cuba breed, then the offspring of that same female must be mated with a bull of that same breed and so on for four or five generations.

When this occurs, the product of that last offspring will be consolidated as a new breed called Siboney de Cuba. As can be seen, obtaining and consolidating a new breed of cattle requires meticulous planning and execution, along with good selection that discards individuals that deviate from the desired theoretical standard. The time that this process can take up to 25 to 30 years.

Summary

The mating system produces changes in the genotype frequencies of populations. Depending on the system used, the frequency of homozygous genotypes will increase or decrease. In populations where random mating is carried out, the offspring will be in Hardy-Weinberg equilibrium.

Matings occur considering the phenotypic similarity or genetic relationships between individuals.

Inbreeding is the mating between individuals that are more closely related than the average of the population to which they belong. Its main effect is the increase in homozygosity at all segregating loci and is one of the most important causes of the decrease in genetic variation within unselected populations.

The measure of inbreeding is the inbreeding coefficient, denoted by **F** and defined as: the probability that two genes at the same locus are identical by descent. This measure is relative to the base population, which must be defined in order to interpret the **F** value.

Inbreeding depression, another effect of inbreeding, is the reduction of the average phenotypic value of traits related to the reproductive capacity or physiological efficiency of animals. This depressive effect is not manifested with equal intensity in all traits. Characters such as fertility, viability, litter size and incubability, among others, show greater sensitivity to inbreeding depression.

Crossbreeding refers to the mating of individuals that are less closely related to each other than the average of the population to which they belong.

Through this mating system, several favorable effects are obtained that together increase productive efficiency.

The presence of heterosis or hybrid vigor, as well as complementarity between breeds, are the most important effects in crossbreeding.

Crossbreeding produces three types of heterosis: individual, maternal and paternal, which can be combined to produce a greater effect on the phenotypic value of the crossed progeny.

The characteristics that exhibit a greater degree of heterosis are those that suffer more intensely from inbreeding depression, thus, reproductive capacity, in general, improves its phenotypic averages in the crossed populations.

It is commonly true that the characters that show a greater degree of inbreeding depression are favored by heterosis and have low inheritance rates. Likewise, the traits less affected by inbreeding depression present a lower amount of heterosis and have medium or high inheritance rates.

There are two main hypotheses for the genetic explanation of hybrid vigor, the theory of dominance and of over-dominance.

The first basically proposes the superiority of the dominant alleles, when the recessive allele is deleterious; and the second considers the superiority of heterozygous genotypes over homozygous ones.

The amount of heterosis in a trait is measurable from the deviation between the average of the reciprocal crosses of the progeny (F_1) and the average of the parental populations.

Complementarity between breeds is another favorable effect that can be obtained in crossed populations. It refers to the ability of two or more breeds to combine well, so that the merit of the offspring for their total productivity is maximized.

The objective of new breeds is to obtain optimal combinations of characteristics that are separately present in the parental populations and that, in addition, are better adapted to the particular conditions of a given environment.

Most of the breeds recognized today come from the crossing of two or more breeds, and in general they present certain advantages, although not all problems are solved by this means.

Chapter 5

Selection systems for dairy cattle

Contents:
Introduction. Dairy cattle selection systems. Traits of economic importance. Fertility. Milk and butter yield. Type and conformation. Selection of cows for breeding. Selection and crossbreeding in dairy cattle. Selection of young bulls. Comprehensive evaluation of breeding stock. Productive indicators to consider animals with dairy biotype.

Introduction

To effectively achieve genetic improvement in any livestock population, it is necessary to use a selection system that takes into account the main production traits that are related to the objectives pursued by the breeder. This chapter provides the basic data necessary for the breeder to choose and develop his indicators as selection criteria to produce bovine milk.

Dairy Cattle Selection Systems

Traits of Economic Importance

The traits of greatest economic importance in dairy cattle are fertility, milk yield, butter yield, type and length of productive life.

Fertility

Normal and consistent reproduction in dairy cattle is of great importance because the lactation period begins when the calf is born.

Estimates of heritability and repeatability for fertility in dairy cattle are very low. These low estimates indicate that most of the observed variation in fertility is due to the environment and, therefore, selection for this trait is not effective.

The greatest improvement within the herd would then come from proper attention to environmental factors such as nutrition, management and disease control.

The fact that estimates of heritability and repeatability for fertility are low does not mean that genes do not affect this trait. This only means that the amount of additive genetic variance affecting fertility is small, and it does not reduce the possibility that a single pair, or at least a small number of pairs of genes with non-additive effects, have an important influence on this trait.

Milk and butter yield

The estimated heritability and repeatability for milk yield and fat percentage are summarized in Table 5-1. The values presented show that milk yield and fat yield heritability are medium to high, so these traits can be genetically improved. Selection for butter percentage should be especially effective, since this trait has a heritability of 60-65 %.

Table 5-1 Heritability and repeatability of milk and butter

Repeatability	Average/%	Range/%
Milk production	53	41-64
Butter production	42	41-43
Butter percentage	68	59-80
Non-fat solids	76	-

Measuring milk and butter production

It is known that several non-genetic factors can cause variations in the production records of dairy cows. Adjusting records for the factors that provoke variations can make selection more effective because superior animals may then be better due to their heredity.

Some of these factors can be corrected by production records for a standard length of time or by using adjustment factors derived from body size data for many animals.

It should be noted that the age of the cows also has an important influence on the amount of milk produced. The peak production of 3-4 year-old cows is considerably lower than that of 6-7 year-old cows. After 9 years of age, cows gradually decrease production.

The number of times a cow is milked is also an important source of variation in milk production. The higher frequency of milkings. This results in the production of more milk and so comparisons between cows that are milked twice daily with those milked three or four times daily are not valid.

Internationally, lactation records for dairy cows of European origin are taken on a 305 days' basis, because this reduces the variation in production records caused by various lactation lengths and because pregnancy has little or no influence on production during a lactation period of that length.

This lactation period is also more desirable, because cows must calve every year and must have a dry period between two successive lactations.

However, in dairy cows obtained from the improved cross between *Bos taurus* and *Bos indicus*, in Cuba for example, the new Siboney breed of Cuba, 240 or 270 days are taken as the basis, which is the length of the effective lactation period in this breed under existing low-input farming conditions.

The dairy and butter-milk register consists of the precise recording of milk production or milk and fat during each lactation period of the producing cow.

This register, to be rigorous, should be kept daily; but in this way it would be incompatible with its practical application. The distance between each two successive controls increases the cause of error; but it is universally established that the monthly control is sufficiently accurate to allow its application without inconvenience.

The technique used in the dairy register comprises the following operations:

1- **Collection of milk samples.** Following the criterion of the monthly interval for a lactation of 300 days, the first sample should be taken for the first time on the seventh day after calving and then monthly until 300 days. The control will be made with the mixture in proportional parts of the quantities of milk obtained in the morning and afternoon milkings: the sum of both quantities constitutes the total to be recorded.

2- **Laboratory analysis.** Using one of the known butyrometry methods, the percentage of milk fat corresponding to the sample is determined. This result is recorded to perform the corresponding calculations.

3- **Calculations.** Once the quantity of milk controlled and converted into the daily average is known, as well as the quantity of fat converted into butter production, the quantity of milk reduced to 4 % fat can be calculated, obtaining a final number that will be comparable with any production from other cows, of different ages and with a milk production of different fat content.

The dairy controller needs to be provided with a portable scale with a force of 20 kg and a sensitivity of 100 g (spring or digital scale), a tared bucket, 100 ml bottles for the samples and a bottle with preservative to add these.

If scales are not available, 10 liter buckets can be used, with a calibration every 500 ml. Mechanical milking equipment allows milk production to be measured in liters at each milking.

In these cases, the weighing of the milk is replaced by its measurement in liters. Although it is not its exact mass, it is accepted that one liter of milk is equivalent to one kg.

Average productive life span

This is another feature of economic importance. It has been observed that the average productive life span of dairy cows is 4 to 6 years.

The reasons for the elimination of 50 % of the cows in a herd have been due to udder problems, low production and reproductive disorders.

Cow longevity is estimated to be 37% heritable. Reproductive efficiency, expressed as the percentage derived from the actual calving interval in days to the ideal of 365 days, had a heritability of 32 %.

The association between the length of productive life span and reproductive efficiency was low to insignificant.

Type and conformation

In dairy cattle, type has a heritability of 25 %. This indicates that only moderate progress could be expected in selection for improvement of this trait.

Type and conformation are valuable because superiority of these traits may help the animal maintain a long and highly productive life.

The most desirable elements are size and mammary gland development, good teat size and placement, limb integrity, and body capacity.

Table 5-2 Indicators of the new dairy breeds of Cuba

Indicator/Breed	HT	M	S	T
Age at puberty/months	15	21,5	21,6	19
Weight at puberty/kg	368	295	311	324
Age at first calving/months	35	36	30	33
Interpartum interval/day	400	383	392	357
Milk production/kg/day	18	8,7	9,8	13
Lactation duration/days	310	263	249	270

Legend: HT = Holstein tropical; M= Mambi; S = Siboney; T= Taino

Selection of cows for breeding

Genetic progress is transmitted from one generation to another through four different pathways:

1. Selection of bulls to produce bulls for the next generation.
2. Selection of females (mothers of breeding stock) to produce bulls for the next generation.
3. Selection of bulls to produce replacement females.
4. Selection of females to produce replacement females.

More than 80 % of genetic progress comes from the first two pathways. In Cuba, the selection of mothers of breeding stock is carried out based on the following criteria:

- Standardized milk production at 3.3 % fat in 244 days and 305 days of lactation.

Let us take as an example the requirements to obtain the status of mother of breeding stock of the Holstein breed. The milk production data will be taken, according to the age at which the female produces in each lactation (Table 5-3).

Table 5-3 Criteria for production of 3.3% standardized milk, in kg

Age years	244 days	305 days
< 3	5 124	6 100
3-4	5 472	6 582
4-5	5 961	7 170
5-6	6 242	7 507
6-7	6 344	7 625
7-8	6 344	7 625

Morphological classification of mothers

Classification by type is basically the comparison of each eligible animal in the herd with the Holstein type closest to the ideal, to arrive at a numerical value. The final value represents the degree of physical perfection obtained and can be expressed in numbers or alphabetically as indicated in Table 5-4.

The final value is the result of four main considerations: general appearance; dairy character; body capacity and mammary system, which contribute with specific value to the final score of the female (Table 5-5).

In addition, the animal is categorized according to its size, due to the importance in genetic improvement of obtaining large animals, capable of high consumption of voluminous feed, mainly grasses (Table 5-6). To reach the category of mother of breeder, it is established as a requirement that the cow obtains the minimum general classification of good.

Table 5-4 Animal score according to its class

Classification	Nomenclature	Points
Excellent	Ex	90 o more
Very good	VG	85-89
More than good	MTG	80-84
Good	G	75-79
Fair	F	65-74
Poor	P	64 or less

Table 5-5 Morphological selection index

Appearance to be classified	Nomenclature	Points
General classification	GC	100
General appearance	GA	30
Dairy character	DC	20
Body capacity	BC	20
Mammary system	MS	30

Table 5-6 Category of the animal according to its size

Size	Nomenclature	Size in cm	Weight (kg)
Large	L	142	645
Medium	M	137-142	560-645
Small	S	137	560

Genetic and phenotypic correlations

Table 5-7 presents some examples of genetic and phenotypic associations found between some productive and morphological traits in dairy cattle, so that they can be used in genetic improvement programs.

Table 5-7 Genetic (Gc) and phenotypic (Pc) correlations in cattle

Characteristics	Gc	Pc
Milk production / Fat production	70,80	+ 0,90
Milk production / Protein production	+ 0,90	+ 0,95
Milk production % fat	- 0,30	- 0,20
Fat production / Protein production	+ 0,90	+ 0,95
Milk production / General appearance	- 0,25	-
Milk production / Body capacity	- 0,20	-

Selection of cows in herds

The trend in modern farms is to impregnate heifers to calve as early as possible and to carry out intensive selection for milk production during the first months of lactation.

Cows that prove to be poor milkers are sold for beef before the end of the first lactation. However, the culling of cows from a herd should preferably be based on all available records as a result of the attention that must be paid to known environmental factors that may influence the various records.

Selection, development and breeding of replacement cows

1- Characteristics in heifers

1) Fertility
    a) Feminine appearance
    b) Calving ease
    c) Maternal ability
    d) Weaning weight
2) Maternal ability
3) Milk production
4) Maternal care
5) Adaptation to the environment

2- Breeding and management program

1) Crossbreeding to exploit hybrid vigor
2) Breed selection including *Bos taurus* and *Bos indicus*
3) Mating season
4) Parasite and disease control

3- Selection of crossbred heifers

A. At weaning

1) Reserve 30 heifers for every 100 cows
2) Selection by: weaning weight and conformation

B. Before the mating period

1) Culling 10 %
   a) For poorer development (weight for age)
   b) Conformation
   c) Femininity

C. After mating - Pregnancy diagnosis

1) Culling: 5-20 %
   a) All opened cows (up to 25 %)
   b) If the number of heifers exceeds 25 %, culling those that had calves with less weight or had stillborn calves (up to 25 %)
   c) Summary: For every 100 cows in the herd
      - Reserve: 30 heifers for replacement
        - Culling: 3 before the breeding season
        - Culling: 5 opened in the first year
        - Culling: 2 that did not wean their calves
        - Culling: 5 opened - second year
      - Remaining: 15 pregnant cows for replacement

4- Development of crossbred heifers

1) Age at first calving - Depends on the breed and its nutritional status

2) So that they give birth at 2-3 years

   a) It is required that from weaning to breeding they receive good grazing with supplements so that they reach a minimum weight of 300 kg at 18-24 months of age
   b) Mate with bulls that produce small calves at birth (zebu or their crossbreds)
   c) Breeding period - short and early. Duration: 60-90 days

3) For calving at 3 to 3.5 years

A. Time of first calving

1) Births should be observed to be attended to in case of dystocia
2) They should be fed properly to maintain growth before and after calving
3) They should reach an average weight of 300 kg before calving

Selection and crossbreeding in dairy cattle

The possibilities of achieving genetic improvement in a dairy cattle population increase with increasing breeding stock size, because progeny testing and selection of bulls can be organized more efficiently than on a small farm.

Progeny testing and selection among bulls

Progeny testing of bulls should be carried out as early as possible to ensure effective selection of tested bulls.

The age at which the bull reaches the end of the test depends on:

a. The age of the young bull when he is capable of producing semen of satisfactory fertility.

b. The time elapsed until enough first lactation records are obtained.

The pattern for continuing to manage young bulls during the test interval varies. In some cases, they provide limited service with AI; sometimes they are rented to other herds as natural breeding bulls, and sometimes they are completely retired from breeding.

Semen can also be collected regularly and stored until the end of the test. Once enough semen for about 50,000 inseminations has been collected and frozen, it could be sent to the slaughterhouse to reduce maintenance costs until the progeny test has been completed.

In the organization of progeny tests there are three important aspects to consider:

a) Testing capacity, i.e. total number of cows with records of their milk production available for test matings.

b) Number of young bulls to be tested each year.

c) Number of daughters with a record of a first lactation needed to carry out the test (group size = n).

Selection of young bulls

The selection of a bull will be based on the merits of his sire and dam, as well as on his own phenotype. The sire will be one of the best bulls available with progeny tests and the dam will be a distinguished cow.

Phenotypic characteristics can be best determined if bulls are raised in large batches on the same farm and subjected to standard feeding and management conditions. Growth rate and feed consumption can then be recorded, and their mating ability and semen quality studied.

Comprehensive evaluation of breeding stock

Morphological selection

Knowledge of the external characteristics of bulls allows us to appreciate their correct conformation and organic integrity, providing us with the basic details to distinguish the best-endowed individuals within the breed and to carry out an intelligent morphological and functional selection.

This method is much more effective in breeds intended for meat production because the conformation of the animal shows its aptitude or gives us more exact details of what it is capable of transmitting to its offspring.

The first point to consider is that the bull is purebred, which is verified by its pedigree and because it meets all the characteristics of its breed.

In summary, when selecting bulls, one does not look for the extremes of any trait. It is best to look for bulls that possess a combination of desirable traits for the genetic improvement of the herd. A selection index can be made for this purpose.

The genetic improvement program on a small scale, that is, in one or several herds, can be carried out as long as there is an adequate correspondence between the genetic potential of milk production of the animals and the feeding and management conditions of the farm.

The breeder must calculate what milk production he can aspire to with the available resources and with the type of animal he has; what he must do to improve the pastures and ensure adequate feeding throughout the year.

Depending on the answers to these questions and the particular conditions of each place, decisions will be made regarding the most appropriate crossbreeding for each case, the use of natural mating or artificial insemination, with duly tested bulls of the selected breed. There are no unique programs, but those that are required, according to the conditions of the population and its environment.

This genetic improvement work is only possible if there is a control system, where the productive behavior of the animals is recorded, since without this information it is impossible to do so.

These systems will be complex depending on the conditions and characteristics of each place, but as simple as they may be, it is indisputable that if they are managed properly, they are a very useful tool for the breeder.

The minimum data required for registration are: Identification, date of birth, name and breed of father and mother, birth weight, weaning weight, age and weight at incorporation, age at first birth, duration of lactation, persistence, milk production per lactation, maternal ability and longevity. Based on the most desired productive and morphological traits, establish a selection index for females.

Productive indicators to consider animals with dairy biotype

The main productive indicators to consider animals with dairy biotype are:

Male

a. Birth weight (from breeder records)
b. Calf weaning weight, kg
c. Age at puberty/months

Female

a. Birth weight (from breeder records)
b. Calf weaning weight, kg
c. Age at first calving, months
d. Duration of lactation, days
e. Milk production (kg/lactation)
f. Fat or butter production (kg/lactation)

Secondary qualitative indicators

a. Maternal ability
b. Ease of calving
c. Docile temperament
d. Average growth rate
e. Fertility and health
f. Longevity

Chapter 6

Selection systems for beef cattle

Contents:
Introduction. Selection systems. Traits of economic importance. Correlations between traits. Bull selection and performance tests. Example of a selection index. Suggestions for an improvement program.

Introduction

In order to effectively achieve genetic improvement of a beef cattle population, it is necessary to use a selection system that takes into account the main productive traits that are related to the objectives pursued by the breeder. This chapter provides the basic data necessary for the breeder to choose and develop his indicators as selection criteria for the quantitative and qualitative improvement of beef production.

Selection systems

The productivity of a breed or crossbreed is based on the kilograms of the final product delivered per unit of time and animal. This is determined by the growth potential of its male offspring and by the reproductive characteristics of its female offspring.

In beef cattle selection programs, these two types of traits are grouped into:

Numerical productivity

Those traits that define the reproductive characteristics of the species and the maternal ability to produce and wean strong and developed calves each year. They are of genetic value for indirect effect

Below are the aspects that determine numerical productivity:

Numerical productivity

Ability to produce and wean a calf

Interval between calvings

Age at calving

Services per gestation

Weight productivity

These are traits that define the characteristics of growth, efficiency in the use of feed and composition of the carcass. They are of genetic value for direct effect.

These are:

> **Weight Productivity**
>
> Pre-weaning growth
>
> Post-weaning growth
>
> Carcass Characteristics

Indirect effect

These are the traits that are manifested indirectly through the behavior of their offspring.

Direct effect

This is the one that is manifested directly in the breeder or in his male offspring.

These are the traits that must be controlled since the selection will be based on this information.

Traits of economic importance that can be used as selection indices

The **DEP** (expected difference between offspring) predict how the future offspring of the listed bulls will behave in each of the production characteristics evaluated. The **DEP** can be positive(+), negative(-) or zero(0), and are expressed in the unit of measurement corresponding to each trait.

The **Prec** (precision) indicates the degree of reliability that can be had in the accompanying **DEP**. A **Prec** close to 1 (one) indicates high reliability, while close to 0 (zero), low reliability. If a sire bull does not leave progeny in 3 or more farms (Rod.), his **Prec** is restricted to a maximum of 0.85. This is valid for any trait evaluated.

1. **GEST:** The gestation length represents the number of days between conception and birth. This EPD predicts the difference in days (more or less) in the gestation length that the progeny of a particular sire bull will have, compared to another. Research indicates that females with shorter gestation intervals have more time to recover and improve their reproductive efficiency. In turn, shorter gestation lengths are associated with lower birth weights and tend to have fewer difficulties at birth.

2. **Birth weight:** This EPD, expressed in kilograms, predicts the capacity of the bull considered to transmit birth weight to his progeny.

- In the example, the offspring of Bull A are expected to weigh on average, 1.2 kilos less than those of Bull B (+1.4 minus + 0.2 = 1.2 Kg). Birth weight is an indicator of calving ease; higher EPDs generally indicate greater calving problems (dystocia).

3. **Weaning weight:** This EPD, expressed in kilos, predicts the ability of the bull considered to transmit growth at weaning to his offspring. All weaning weights analyzed were adjusted to 205 days and by age of the mother.

    - In the example, the offspring of Bull A are expected to weigh on average, 3.4 kilos less than those of Bull B (+8.6 minus +5.2 = 3.4 Kg).

4. **Milk production:** This EPD indicates the dairy ability that a bull transmits to his daughters, measured through the weaning weight of his grandsons.

    - In the example, Bull A's daughters provide an extra amount of milk that allows them to wean offspring that weigh 7.8 kilos more, on average, than those born to Bull B (+6.7 minus -1.1 = 7.8 Kg). It is also important to note that each daughter also transmits to her offspring, along with these genes for milk, the genes for growth from her father.

5. **Final weight:** This EPD, expressed in kilos, predicts the capacity of the bull considered to transmit growth to his offspring, measured as weight at 18 months.

- In the example, Bull A's offspring will weigh on average, at one and a half years of age, 5.6 kilos more than Bull B's (+14.9 minus +9.3 = 5.6 Kg).

6. **Scrotal circumference (S.C.):** This EPD, expressed in centimeters and adjusted to 18 months, predicts the bull's ability to transmit this characteristic to his offspring.

    - Our example indicates that the offspring of Bull A will have on average, at 18 months of age, 1.2 cm more scrotal circumference than those of Bull B (+1.2 minus +0.0 = 1.2 cm). Remember that scrotal circumference is one of the best predictors of fertility, since it is associated with the quantity of semen produced by the bull and with the age at which his offspring enter puberty (sexual precocity); higher EPDs mean that the offspring will reach sexual maturity earlier.

7. **Height:** This EPD, expressed in centimeters and adjusted to 18 months, is very important when you must choose, for example, between two bulls with the same final weight EPD, in order to avoid increasing body size beyond what is desired.

8. **Back fat thickness (DFT):** This EPD, expressed in millimeters and adjusted to 18 months, predicts the bull's ability to transmit greater or lesser back fat thickness (DFT) to its offspring, depending on whether its value is positive or negative, respectively.

9. **Hip fat thickness (HFT):** This EPD, expressed in millimeters and adjusted to 18 months, predicts the bull's ability to transmit greater or lesser hip fat thickness (HFT) to its offspring, depending on whether its value is positive or negative, respectively.

10. **Dorsal L. Area (D.L.A):** This EPD, expressed in square centimeters and adjusted to 18 months, predicts the bull's ability to transmit a greater or lesser area of the L. dorsi muscle to its offspring, depending on whether its value is positive or negative, respectively.

11. **Intermuscular Fat (GI):** This EPD, expressed as a percentage and adjusted to 18 months, predicts the bull's ability to transmit a greater or lesser percentage of intramuscular fat (%GI) to its offspring, depending on whether its value is positive or negative, respectively.

12. **Retail Cut (%CM):** The percentage of retail cuts (%CM) is a composite EPD that mainly combines information on weight at the time of ultrasound measurement (PM), the area of L. dorsi (ALD) and the thickness of dorsal fat (EGD). It predicts the difference in kilos of retail cuts that the offspring of a particular sire bull would give on average, with respect to another.

Heritability of the main traits of economic importance

Birth weight

An h^2 of 0,30 to 0,40 has been found, and this trait may be due to selection.

Pre-weaning growth

A mean value of 0,22 has been observed for this trait. The low heritability of this trait is of little importance since most of the growth in intensive meat production occurs in fattening lots.

Weaning weight

This trait is useful for evaluating differences in maternal capacity and for measuring deficiencies in the growth potential of calves. An average heritability value of 0,27 has been found, which is relatively low.

Post-weaning growth

The growth index is important due to its high association with gain efficiency, its high heritability (0,50) and its high correlation with other traits of economic importance.

Carcass traits

Most of the traits included in carcass merit are influenced by many genes. Carcass measurements can be taken when animals are of the same age (constant age) or when they have the same weight (constant weight).

From the results presented in the following table it can be deduced that these traits can be genetically improved.

Table 6-1 Heritability of some carcass traits

Traits	h^2
Carcass weight per day of age	0,40 - 0,50
Edible meat/ %	0,40
Prime meat/ %	0,30
L. dorsali area	0,25 - 0,40

Reproductive traits: have very low heritability coefficients.

Table 6-2 Pre-weaning growth traits

Pre-weaning grow traits	h^2
Birth weight	0,30 a 0,40
Gain	0,22 a 0,40
Post-weaning growth	0,27

Table 6-3 Heritability of some traits of productive efficiency

Heritability of Traits	
Conversion	0,40
Maturity rate	0,40
Weight at maturity	0,50
Consumption	0,45

Trait correlations

Cold carcass weight is positively correlated with edible meat content and kidney fat and negatively correlated with bone content.

Total edible meat content is positively correlated with prime meat quantity and yield. Carcass weight is a good indicator of yield and allows predicting L. dorsi area, total edible meat and bone content.

For preliminary general selection, attention should be paid to the following aspects:

   a. Conformation
   b. Temperament
   c. Hardiness
   d. Breeding ability and fertility potential
   e. Superiority of body mass over 20% of the population average

Bull selection and performance testing

Bull selection

Herd genetic improvement requires a system to measure economic characteristics in each animal and use this information in the selection of bulls and cows of the next generation. This system is called performance testing.

A. A complete test should include:

1) Birth weight
2) Weaning weight
3) Post-weaning weight gain, measured on the farm or at a test center
4) Permanent identification of each individual and data record
5) Adjustment of weights for sex, age, age of dam, season or date of birth and contemporary group
6) Carcass merit measures
7) Reproductive trait measures

B. Rules in performance testing:

1) Equal treatment for all calves
2) Written performance records
3) Comparison within calves of similar age and adjust weights for differences in age and age of dam
4) Purchase calves or young bulls that come from herds with a very similar environment to yours

Characteristics of each sire purpose in order of importance

A. For first-calf cows consider:

1) Calving ease
    a. Low birth weight
    b. Poor muscle development
2) Fertility and health

3) Docile temperament

4) Low growth rate

B. To produce replacement cows, consider:

1) Maternal ability

2) Average growth rate

3) Fertility and health

4) Docile temperament

5) Ease of calving

6) Merit of the breed

In summary, bull selection does not seek the extremes of any trait. It is best to look for bulls that possess a combination of desirable traits for the genetic improvement of the herd. A selection index must be made for this purpose.

The small-scale genetic improvement program, that is, in one or several herds, can be carried out as long as there is an adequate correspondence between the genetic potential for meat production of the animals and the feeding and management conditions of the farm.

The breeder must calculate what meat production he can aspire to with the available resources and with the type of animal he has; what he must do to improve the pastures and ensure adequate feeding throughout the year.

Depending on the answer obtained to these questions and the particular conditions of each place, decisions will be made regarding the most appropriate crossbreeding for each case, the use of natural mating or artificial insemination, with duly tested bulls of the selected breed. There are no unique programs, but those that are required, according to the particular conditions of the population and its environment.

This genetic improvement work is only possible if there is a *control system*, where the productive behavior of the animals is recorded, since without this information it is impossible to do it.

These systems will be more or less complex depending on the conditions and characteristics of each place, but as simple as they are, it is indisputable that if they are managed properly, they are a very useful tool for the breeder.

Behavior test

A behavior test consists of measuring certain traits in the living animal, such as growth evaluation, food conversion, daily gain, reproductive indicators, etc.

Advantage

The main advantage of this test is that it allows the evaluation of the animal at a much earlier age than the progeny test. In this way, the interval between generations is reduced and it becomes possible to use the bull during its most productive years.

Although the behavior test is less exact than the progeny test, the former allows for greater intensity of selection.

Disadvantage

The disadvantage of the behavior test is that it is not applicable to those traits that cannot be measured in the living animal, such as carcass characteristics or those with low heritability.

Testing systems

Animals may be tested by:

    a. Fixed period system

    b. Age-based system

    c. Specific weight system

    d. Combined system (age-based to constant weight)

In any performance test animals should be selected on the basis of their superiority in the trait(s) desired to be obtained in the progeny.

Feeding systems

The objective of any testing system should be to evaluate, as quickly and efficiently as possible, the genetic differences between animals in terms of their phenotypic expression.

The greater the environmental variation between the bulls being tested due to variations in feeding, the more difficult it will be to achieve this objective since the heritability of the trait is reduced.

Everything seems to indicate that a complete diet based on concentrates is the most appropriate because:

1- The daily increase will be limited only by the animal's growth potential
2- The diet will be the same for all animals and even comparisons between years will be valid
3- This diet facilitates management and increases the accuracy when recording data

Housing

Housing should be individual because the group system prevents measuring consumption and conversion, which means that valuable information is lost. Straw bedding should not be used because the animals consume it and it can alter the results.

In any test, it is necessary to take into account the homogeneity of the experimental group to prevent a dominant animal in the social hierarchy from affecting profits to such an extent that an animal with high genetic potential appears inferior to another of poorer quality, due to its docility or smaller age or size.

The most commonly used selection criteria are:

a) Initial and final weight

b) Daily gain

c) Weight for age

d) Feed consumption

e) Conversion

It is advisable to weigh the animals periodically in order to be able to draw up their growth curve, as well as to accustom them to routine handling.

The more reduced the criteria for selection, the faster the progress of any of them will be. The most important trait in meat production is the amount of edible meat produced per unit of feed consumed.

The fact that weight for age is used as a selection criterion in some cases is because it is considered the best measure of growth rate, in addition, this trait is highly correlated (r= 0.71) with daily gain, which makes the effects of compensatory growth minimal.

The pasture performance test (PPT)

This is a system that every livestock breeder should know. It guarantees the selection of the parents of the next generation, a fundamental pillar in any genetic improvement program.

The PPT evaluates animals of the same sex under uniform farming conditions to identify breeding animals.

It is important that when purchasing semen from AI establishments or when acquiring breeding bulls, you do so with the guarantee that the animals are certified by the performance test on pasture and progeny.

If a scale for larger animals is not available to measure the live weight of animals, I recommend printing and using the conversion table of live weight according to the size of the thoracic circumference, which appears in Table 6-4.

For this, a measuring tape, preferably made of cloth, 200 cm long, is used and placed around the thorax, as indicated in Figure 6-1. The tape should be placed, but not tightened, to avoid measurement errors. In fattened animals, the tape should be placed at the thoracic insertion point of the hump.

To avoid errors in judgment, the measurements should always be made by the same person, preferably the breeder.

Although the conversion of chest circumference into live weight is not exact for all bovine breeds, these measurements will serve as useful data for the selection purposes that are required, since the most important thing is the comparison between individuals.

Example of a Selection Index

Beef cattle are rarely selected on a single trait, so the economic value or net worth of an animal is determined by several traits.

In a study in the USA, weaning weight was found to be the most accurate trait for selecting the rate of gain expressed in a herd.

A simple index of considerable accuracy, in addition to weaning weight, was I = WW + 72GR, where WW is the weaning weight and GR is the rate of gain in the finishing area.

Another, more complicated index:

I = 0.58WW + 18.64DG - 0.73F - 5.87E, where WW is weaning weight; DG, the daily gain in the fattening area, with a short period between weaning and the start of the test, to bring the animals to a full fattening cycle, F, the number of days to bring each animal to a minimum weight for slaughter; and E, the amount of feed per pound of gain.

To illustrate the calculation of such an index, I offer an example taken from Lasley (1973).

Selection Index

WW = 400 lbs
GR = 2.5 lbs
F = 200 days
E = 7.5 lbs

The calculated index would be:

I = 0.58(400) + 18.64(2.50) - 0.73(200) - 5.87(7.5)
I = 232 + 46.6 - 146 - 44.03
I = 88.57

Note: 1 kg = 2,2 lbs 1 lb. = 460 g
Legend:
WW weaning weight
GR gain rate
DG daily gain
F equals number of days for full fattening
E equals amount of feed for daily gain

This index serves as an example to show how some important factors can be considered in constructing an index to aid in selection for maximum genetic improvement.

It may or may not be applicable to the selection of beef cattle in the areas of a given region, or it may be modified or adjusted to the characteristics of the farming system in question.

Fig. 6-1 How to place the measuring tape to measure the chest circumference in a cow

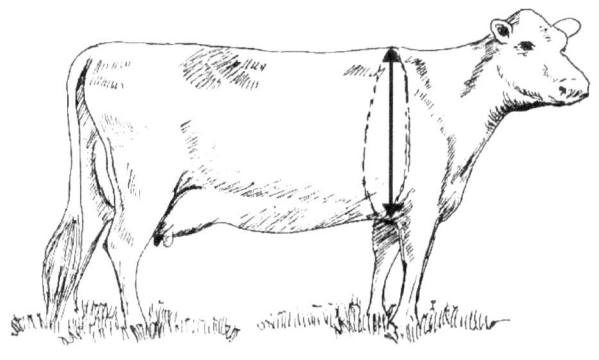

Table 6-4 Conversion of thoracic perimeter to live weight

TP	LW	TP	LW	TP	LW	TP	LW
60	28	95	80	130	181	165	358
61	28	96	82	131	184	166	368
62	29	97	85	132	188	167	378
63	30	98	87	133	192	168	388
64	31	99	90	134	196	169	399
65	32	100	92	135	200	170	408
66	33	101	95	136	204	171	420
67	34	102	97	137	208	172	430
68	35	103	99	138	212	173	440
69	36	104	101	139	217	174	450
70	37	105	104	140	222	175	459
71	38	106	106	141	227	176	467
72	38	107	109	142	232	177	473
73	39	108	111	143	237	178	477
74	40	109	114	144	242	179	480
75	41	110	116	145	247	180	483
76	42	111	119	146	252	181	486
77	43	112	121	147	257	182	489
78	45	113	123	148	262	183	492
79	47	114	126	149	267	184	495
80	49	115	129	150	272	185	498
81	50	116	132	151	276	186	501
82	52	117	136	152	280	187	503
83	54	118	139	153	284	188	506
84	56	119	142	154	288	189	509
85	57	120	146	155	292	190	512
86	59	121	149	156	296	191	515
87	61	122	153	157	301	192	518
88	63	123	156	158	306	193	521
89	65	124	160	159	312	194	524
90	67	125	164	160	318	195	527
91	69	126	167	161	324	196	530
92	71	127	170	162	331	197	533
93	74	128	174	163	339	198	536
94	77	129	177	164	348	199	539

Legend:
Thoracic perimeter = TP
Live weight = LW

Suggestions for a selection and improvement program

1. Identify all animals with a tattoo on the inside of the ear, a metal clip, plastic art, or any other means that will allow permanent identification of the animal.
2. Record the exact date of birth of each calf, tattoo at birth, and record the calf and cow numbers.
3. Obtain a record of weanlings and weights and correct calf weights for age of dams and age and sex of calf.
4. Retain replacement heifers from those with higher weaning weights and better conformation.
5. Cull cows that after one or two calves give birth to weak calves that are lighter than the average for the herd. Cull on the basis of records and not just type.
6. Weigh and record heifers again at approximately 18 months of age to obtain information on post-weaning gain rates and on group records of bulls, as well as information on the gaining ability of calves from different cows. Discard those heifers with undesirable types or gains or with obviously undesirable traits.
7. Breed all male calves that are superior from the standpoint of type and weaning weight. If they cannot be bred individually, do so as a group, but give all animals equal feeding opportunities. Feed them for at least 150 days and at the end of that period, calculate the efficiency of gain rate and score by type and conformation. Sort bulls by the traits of greatest economic importance and retain the best for breeding purposes.

8. When purchasing bulls from a herd, obtain those from a herd where records of the above types are maintained. Obtain the best bull possible based on type and rate of gain efficiency at the end of the feeding trial. Select a bull from the herd whose dam had a lifetime record of producing a calf each year with type and weaning weight above the population average.

9. If the farm has the conditions for it, introduce artificial insemination and purchase semen from proven bulls of the breed you have decided to use in your improvement program.

Chapter 7

Breeding systems for buffalos

Contents:
Introduction. Peculiarities of the species *Bos bubalis*. Zoological classification. Some behavioral traits of water buffalos. Categories. Swamp buffalos or Carabao. Morphological characteristics. Bufalipso. Morphological characteristics. Basic requirements for the selection of dairy buffalos. Selection of parent buffalos. Selection system for replacement.

Introduction

For the genetic improvement of any buffalo population, a selection system must be used that takes into account the main productive traits that are related to the objectives pursued by the breeder. This chapter provides the basic data available for the breeder to choose and develop his indicators as selection criteria to increase the milk and meat production of his buffalo herd**s**

Peculiarities of the species *Bos bubalos bubalis*

Zoological classification

Order: Artiodactyla

Suborder: Ruminants

Family: Bovids

Subfamily: *Bubalinae*

Species: *Bos Bubalo bubalis*

Subspecies: *Bubalus bubalis carabanensis*

- The world population of buffalo is estimated at 150 million heads and India is the main producer.

- There are 19 breeds of buffalo, the most economically important of which are:

    - Mediterranean, Murrah, Nili-Ravi, Jafrabadi and Carabao.

- Although the river buffalo (*Bos bubalo bubalis*) has 50 chromosomes and the swamp buffalo (*Bos bubalo carabanensis*) 48, the offspring are viable; However, 98 % of the males of the first F_1 generation are sterile, unlike the females, which are fertile.

- The F_2, F_3 and subsequent offspring, which are part of the Bufalipso type absorption program, are fertile in both sexes.

The advantages that are pointed out to the buffalo species with respect to the bovine are the following:

Reproductive capacity, which makes it profitable in any environment

- The climate-soil-plant-buffalo relationship is more effective, since the buffalo makes more efficient use of low quality pastures and adapts better to diverse environments.

- Its digestive system allows it to make better use of food.

- It requires a minimum of investment for its exploitation.

- They are docile, rustic and long-lived.

- They produce milk and meat of excellent quality.

- The leather can be used for the same purposes as that of the bovine.

- They are resistant to tropical diseases and have low mortality.

Some behavioral traits of water buffaloes

In order to properly manage, exploit and select buffaloes, it is necessary for the breeder to know the most important peculiarities of their behavior.

Reproductive

Well-fed buffaloes reach puberty between 15 months and 18 months of age, but are incorporated into breeding at 22-24 months, when they have reached a weight of 375 kg.

The sexual activity of this species is seasonal, so the highest frequency of heat occurs in the winter season (September-January), when the days are somewhat shorter and the nights somewhat longer, that is, on days with less light intensity. Due to this, 90 % of births occur in the months of July to October. The duration of gestation averages 300 days, with a range of variation of 293-318 days.

In herds, it is recommended to use only one father buffalo for every 30 buffaloes. In this way, fights between males are avoided and the paternity of the offspring can be easily recognized.

Parent buffalos over five years old that become aggressive and difficult to handle should be separated from the herd.

Strong gregarious instinct

They always remain grouped together, unlike cattle. This behavior makes it easier to stay and lead the animals to the desired areas.

Temperament and the presence of man

Despite their rusticity, buffalo cattle require more human presence than cattle. The absence or prolonged absence of collections and handling in extensive herds can make some animals difficult to handle.

This means that docility depends on the work carried out by the breeders. They are, by nature, shy and easily frightened, so they must be led calmly and patiently; the use of dogs, rough treatment and shouting make their handling more difficult and their training more arduous.

Longevity

This is one of the most appreciated characteristics of buffaloes. The average biological lifespan of a buffalo is 20-25 years. It is influenced by its adaptive capacity and resistance to diseases.

Wild buffaloes

Swamp buffaloes or Carabao and their F_1 and F_2 crossbreeds are very nervous and prone to form wild buffaloes, that is, to escape and hide in wild groups, avoiding any encounter with man.

Wild buffaloes become predators of all kinds of crops, making them undesirable, as they harm the vegetable production of farmers.

Coexistence between parent buffaloes

As they get older, peaceful coexistence between parent buffaloes becomes more difficult due to problems with the social hierarchy.

To avoid fights, parent buffaloes must be separated and the best one selected to perform the mating. In extensive herds, males must be grouped by age.

Roaming Habit

They are very attached to their place of origin, when they adopt an area it is easy to retain them. When they move to another place, it is necessary to lock them up at night, until they adapt. Generally during this period of the day, they move to return to their place of origin or look for new areas.

Containment

Buffalo are well controlled by barbed wire fences or electric fences. They respect electric fences more than cattle, but it has been proven that the best fence is the food they have in their areas.

They have a strong survival instinct and if they run out of food they will break any type of fence. This is one of the reasons why they walk incessantly and destroy fences and crops. They are not tolerant of hunger.

Water and shade

They need sufficient drinking water to drink and cool off, as well as shade, because they are very sensitive to the effects of intense sunlight.

This is because they have very few sweat glands that allow them to dissipate heat. In addition, the black color of their coat favors greater absorption of sunlight.

Cooling

Buffalo prefer to cool off in wallows, which they often prepare themselves. They can stay in them for up to five hours when the air temperature and solar irradiation are high.

Instinctively, they select areas of clean water to drink, others to wallow in and others to defecate.

Water can come from reservoirs, rivers, ponds and swamps. The wallows they create help to eliminate ectoparasites from their skin.

Coat and skin

In the tropics, their skin has little hair. Calves are born with hair, but they lose it with age. The skin of the buffalo is twice as thick and heavy as that of the cattle (36 vs.18 kg).

Hardiness

They are very hardy and adaptable to different ecosystems. They have a better capacity than cattle to use low-quality pastures and forage.

Milk quality

The content of buffalo milk is higher in fat, proteins and mineral salts than that of cattle. To produce 1 kg of cheese, 12 liters of cow's milk are required, but only 8 liters of buffalo milk. To produce 1 kg of butter, 20 liters of cow's milk are needed, and only 14 liters of buffalo milk.

Table 7-1 Buffalo subspecies

Subspecies	Characteristics	Location	Objectives
River	Black or dark grey colour Slightly curled or straight horns Prefer to wallow in clean waters Have 50 chromosomes	India Egypt Europe Latin America	Milk Production Meat as a by-product
Swamp	Purple-grey colour Solid horns laid back Have 48 chromosomes	Philippines Part of India	Work Meat production Milk as a by-product

Categories

The categories that participate in the zootechnical flow are:

Table 7-2 Categories of zootechnical flow

Calf Buffalo	From birth to 12 months
Yearlings Buffalo	Between 12 and 18 months of age
Female Buffalo	Older than 18 months that have not given birth
Male Buffalo	Males between 18-24 months of age
Mother Buffalo	From the first birth
Father Buffalo	Older than 24 months dedicated to fatherhood

Swamp Buffalo or Carabao

Morphological characteristics

This is the main type of buffalo in the Philippines and India and is used as a working animal in rice fields and for traction. In the state of Para and on Marajo Island in Brazil, it is used for meat production.

Coat Color

They are brownish gray, with white spots on the legs, forehead and neck (in the form of a collar). These wrist bands and collar are observed in crossbreeds of river and swamp buffalo. Much of the body is hairless or has stiff and very short hair.

Head

The forehead is flat, the eyes are prominent, the face is short and the snout is wide. The horns are very long and flattened, and they curve backwards, with the tips very far apart, reaching up to 1.2 m maximum separation between one tip and the other.

Body

Their body is short and their belly is wide, they are compact and solid, with noticeable meaty features. The neck is relatively long, the withers and rump are prominent. Their limbs and tail are short. The udder is small and displaced backwards.

A distinctive feature is that they do not have sexual dimorphism, that is, there are no marked phenotypic differences between males and females. However, males are usually heavier than females (600-700 vs 450-500 kg).

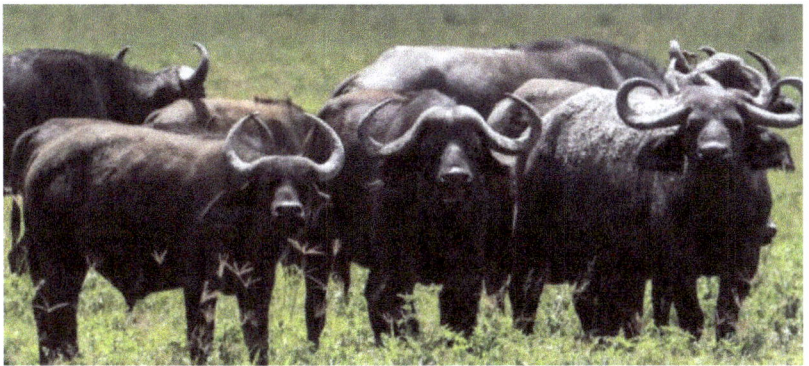

Fig. 7-1. Swamp Buffalo or Carabao

Bufalipso

The Bufalipso river buffalo of Trinidad and Tobago is the product of crossbreeding with the Muraah, Mediterranean Black, Jafrabadi, Nili-Rabi and Carabao buffalo breeds, given that they have some light-colored markings on their legs and neck, typical of the Carabao.

The buffalos of Trinidadian origin have the disadvantage of having some recessive genes that cause albinism.

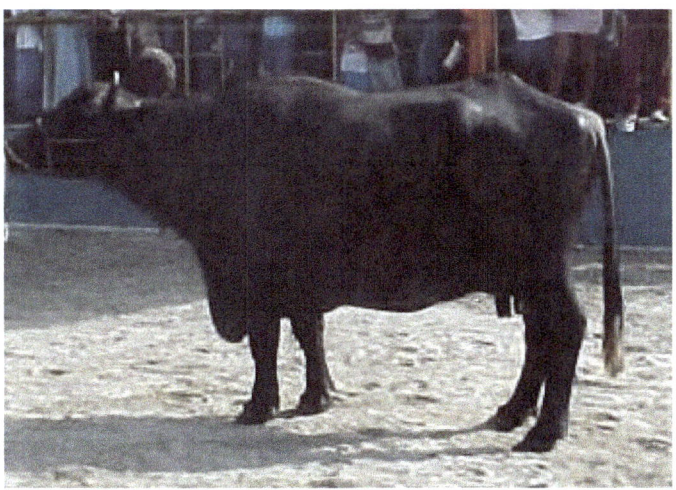

Fig. 7-2 Bufalipso out of water

Morphological characteristics

Coat colour

The coat colour is black or grey.

Head

The head has a long, narrow face and long hairs that are sparse on the lower edge of the jaw. Medium horns, pointing backwards and to the sides, with the tips closed upwards and inwards, forming a half moon.

Body

It is a corpulent animal, 1.8 m tall. The chest is deep and the abdomen is voluminous. The tail is short, but reaches the hock because it is set low.

In general, it is a compact, muscular and deep animal. The udder is medium-sized, well formed. The average live weight of the adult male is 700-800 kg and that of the female 600 kg.

Zootechnical characteristics

In Cuba, the average milk production obtained has been 931.4 kg, in 250 days of lactation, which is equivalent to a daily average of 3.7 kg. The yield in the carcass is 55 %. In fattening pens, at 18 months they can reach weights of 480 kg. Under grazing conditions, at 26 months they can weigh up to 500 kg.

Basic requirements for the selection of dairy buffaloes

1) **Identification:** This is done by tattooing the inside of the ear after birth, branding at weaning and the placement of earrings at incorporation.

2) **Records:** It is essential to control all events, for which a system of records is designed that is easy to keep at the dairy level. This allows for precise selection and maintenance of the history of the herd, quantifying the improvements that are made each year. Control of paternity is essential.

3) **Control of milk weighing:** A system must be designed for buffaloes under a suckling system in which at least two weightings are carried out per month, which are controlled in the dairy itself.

4) **High-producing buffaloes:** Based on milk control and knowledge of their identification and reproductive behavior, high-producing buffaloes are selected, which are those that produce the greatest amount of milk per lactation within the dairy. Their female offspring are protected as replacements for the worst buffaloes and the males as future father buffaloes for the dairy itself or for use in other dairy farms and in the absorption herds.

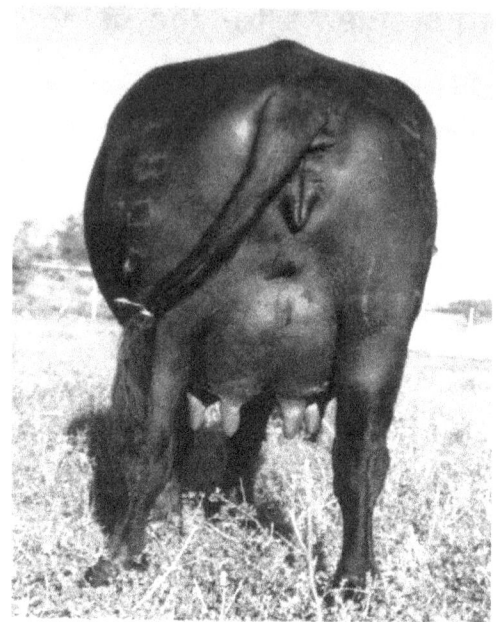

Fig. 7-3 Dairy Buffalo

To achieve good profitability in dairies with 30 buffaloes, the following indicators must be met:

1) More than 100 liters of milk daily with 90 % of the buffaloes being milked.

2) More than 4 liters per day per buffalo in milking.

3) Less than 2 % mortality of calves.

4) More than 90 % birth rate.

5) Replace every year the 4-5 lowest buffaloes in milk production and those that did not give birth.

6) Interval between births, less than 380 days.

7) Duration of lactation between 230 to 250 days.

In addition, in herds of animals in development and fattening, the following factors must be combined:

1) Incorporation into reproduction at 20 to 22 months, with no less than 340 kg of live weight.
2) Age of slaughter of males less than 24 months, with a weight of 450 kg.

Selection of parent buffalos

The selection of the breeding male is done in a similar way to that of cattle already explained in chapters 5 and 6.

Selection systems for replacement

In each herd, the conditions will be created, whenever feasible, to breed the necessary number of females to guarantee replacement.

1) **Selection at weaning:** Daughters of high producers that show growth in accordance with age.
2) **Selection at 12 months of age:** Those females with less development compared to their contemporaries are discarded.
3) **Selections at 15 and 18 months of age:** They will be more rigorous and with the same selection criteria as those applied at 12 months. The latter defines the move to the category of *Female Buffalo*.
4) **Incorporation into reproduction:** They must meet the age and weight requirements (22-24 months and 375 kg). Any *Female Buffalo* that does not become pregnant at the end of the mating stage is subject to discard.

Chapter 8

Selection systems for sheep and goats

Contents:
Introduction. Selection. Traits of economic importance. Fertility. Weaning weight. Post-weaning gain. Type and conformation. Carcass. Obtaining and calculating indicators of productive interest. Selection index. Data needed to create selection indices for males of meat breeds. Selection criteria for females' improvement. Selection criteria for improving dairy males.

Introduction

Sheep and goats are multipurpose animals that produce meat, milk, skin, hair and manure for organic fertilizer for crops. They can consume a greater quantity of food per unit of weight and produce, in turn, more milk per unit of live weight.

- They digest fiber more efficiently, especially with poor diets.

- Their feeding behavior makes them flexible in the selection of diets to satisfy their nutritional requirements (browsing and consumption of a wide variety of plants, etc.). The conversion of consumed food to milk is favorable, although its conversion to meat is lower. However, due to their greater prolificacy, the amount of meat they produce per unit of time is greater. The chemical composition of goat's milk is very similar to that of women and is better tolerated by children with lactose intolerance. In addition, exquisite cheese is produced with it. Other products they produce are their skin, hair and fecal matter as organic fertilizer. Goats represent an alternative for controlling undesirable bushes and weeds in the country.

Selection

One of the main causes of the poor use, diffusion and development of sheep and goat livestock is the inadequate application of technologies in their breeding and an overvaluation of the rusticity of these species. For this reason, there is a deep-rooted tendency to confuse rustic animals, and treat them as wild animals that do not require care, which undermines the directed selection to achieve the genetic improvement of these species.

For these reasons, the genetic improvement of sheep and goat livestock in the tropics is a primary objective, which must be fulfilled, due to the strategic importance of increasing the production of foods with high biological value, such as milk and meat, which are in high demand by the population.

Traits of economic importance

The traits of economic importance in sheep and goats are those related to the production of meat and milk that are necessary for the consumer population.

Due to the productive similarity of these two species, these traits will be discussed only by looking at the type of production.

Fertility

Both species have seasonal reproductive activity, although some breeds may have two lambs per year under good farming conditions.

The number of lambs weaned per sow is one of the most important factors determining the productive efficiency of the animal.

Lamb and kid production varies according to farming conditions and between different breeds. Sows reared under farm conditions are more prolific than those reared freely. This is due to the better level of nutrition they generally find on farms. Twin births in sheep are desirable because a sheep that weans twins produces 15 to 20 kg more meat than one that weans one.

As with other species, fertility has a very low heritability. Therefore, most of the phenotypic variation is due to environmental factors and proper attention to these can increase the number of births.

Weaning weight

For selection purposes, the age of 120 days is used for weaning lambs. Weaning weight in ewes has a 43 % repeatability. Therefore, if environmental conditions remain unchanged, culling ewes that wean lambs with low weights will increase the average weaning weight of the total flock.

Weaning weight in ewes has about 33 % heritability. Thus, selection for this trait will result in some improvement, although it may be slower than for post-weaning gain or some other traits.

Lambs can be weighed when they reach 120 days, or weaning weight can be corrected for this age.

The correction is made by multiplying the average daily gain from birth to weaning age by 120 and adding this product to the birth weight.

Twin weights can be adjusted to a single lamb basis by multiplying the adjusted 120-day weight by the factor 1.0529; for triplets the factor is 1.0923.

Post-weaning gain

The average rate of gain on dry feed lots in sheep has been found to have a high heritability, so selection for mass to improve this trait should be effective. Lamb body weight has an average heritability of 40-45 %, which is high, with high repeatability.

Yearling ewes that weigh more also wean heavier lambs and produce heavier fleeces, so selection for this trait could be effective and desirable.

Type and conformation

As with other farm ruminants, desirable type and conformation in sheep and goats should also be given due attention and only those that meet breed standards and are free from physical and functional defects should be selected.

A system of selection and breeding called "*corrective mating*" has been used successfully.

Ewes that are highly productive but have some undesirable trait can be mated to a ram that is especially outstanding in the trait in which those ewes are inferior.

Often this corrects the deficiency in a single mating. This method of mating, which has been shown to be effective, could be used to improve many undesirable traits.

Carcass

As in cattle, almost all carcass traits are highly heritable in sheep and goats. By selecting from proven parents (progeny testing), or genomic selection, carcass weight, fat content, and meat tenderness can be improved.

Genetic correlations between productive traits

The genetic correlations between milk and meat production traits in sheep and goats are very similar to those in cattle, discussed in chapters 6 and 7, and respond to the same principles of polygenic inheritance.

Obtaining and calculating some indicators of productive interest

- **For weight at different ages**

  Age at weaning/days (AW)

  AW = Date at Weaning - Date of birth

- **Average pre-weaning daily gain/g (AWDG)**

  $$AWDG = \frac{(WW-BW)}{DBW}$$

  Where:
  WW = Weaning weight
  BW = Birth weight
  DBW = Days elapsed between both weighing

- **Adjusted weaning weight/kg (AWW)**

Lambs can be weighed when they reach 120 days, but the weaning weight can be corrected for this age. The correction is made by multiplying the average daily gain from birth to weaning age by 120 and adding this product to the birth weight.

Twin weights can be adjusted on a single lamb basis by multiplying the adjusted 120-day weight by the factor 1.0529; for triplets the factor is 1.0923.

$$AWW = \frac{(WW-WB)}{AW} \times AAW + WB$$

Where:
- WW = Weight at weaning
- WB = Weight at birth
- AW = Individual age at weaning/days
- AAW = Average age at weaning/days

- **Average daily gain for different periods/g (ADG)**

$$ADG = \frac{(FW-IW)}{DBW}$$

Where:
- FW = Final weight
- IW = Initial weight
- DBW = Days elapsed between both weighing

- **Weight for age (WA)**

$$WA = Live\ weight/Age/days$$

For reproduction

- **Age at first calving (AFC)**

  AFC = Date of first calving − Date of birth

- **Calving interval**

  CI = Date of last calving − Date of previous calving

- **Fertility percentage**

  $$\text{Fertility} = \frac{\text{Total females calved}}{\text{Total females exposed}} \times 100$$

- **Prolificacy percentage**

  $$\text{Prolificacy} = \frac{\text{Total calves born}}{\text{Total females calved}} \times 100$$

Selection index

Several indices can be used for selection purposes depending on the breeder's goals.

One index to measure sheep productivity is the lamb's weaning weight divided by the mother sheep's body weight.

Example: If the weaned twin lambs weighed 45 kg and the mother 50 kg, the index would be:

$$\frac{45}{50} = 0{,}9$$

Data needed to create selection indices for males of meat breeds

1) Morphological evaluation
2) Birth weight
3) Weaning weight
4) Daily gain
5) Feed conversion
6) Prolificacy
7) Carcass yield
8) Carcass weight
9) Meat quality

Selection criteria for females' improvement

1) That it meets the morphological standards of the breed.
2) That it has a body development in accordance with its age and sex.
3) That it is the daughter of multiple births.
4) That its parents have good pedigrees.
5) That it has good milk or meat production.
6) That it is docile and has good maternal ability.
7) That it weans its healthy and robust offspring.

Selection criteria for improving dairy males

1) Comply with the morphological patterns of the breed.
2) Have no physical or functional defects
3) Have been born from a multiple birth.
4) Come from high milk producing mothers: It is advisable to consider the corresponding lactations between the 2nd and 3rd birth (maximum peak production).
5) That during weaning it has reached daily gains greater than 100g/day.
6) That its reproductive system is healthy and functional and with acceptable mating capacity.

Bibliography

Abney, M. (2008): *Identity by descent estimation and mapping of qualitative traits in large, complex pedigree.* Genetics. 179:1577-1590.

Alba, L. O. y Fleites, R. (1974): *Valores testiculares en toros cebú de 3 a 6 años, producción de semen y su relación con las medidas testiculares.* IV Jornada de Ciencias Veterinarias. Facultad de Ciencias Agropecuarias. Universidad Central de L.V. Cuba.

Alba, L. O. (1977): *Algunos aspectos del comportamiento reproductivo de los toros Brahman americano incorporados al programa de inseminación artificial en Cuba.* Tesis en opción al grado de Doctor en Ciencias Veterinarias. Universidad de Veterinaria de Brno, República Checa.

Alba L.O., Castellanos Odmara, Silveira E. (2006): *Comportamiento sexual de toros en la sala de monta según las técnicas de refrenamiento.* REDVET 7(2):12-25.

Alba, L.O. (2019): *Peculiaridades de la morfometría ovárica y cervical: del ganado Bos indicus y de sus cruzamientos con Bos Taurus.* 1ra Ed. Libro electrónico en PDF. Editorial Universitaria ISBN 978-959-16-4319-3. La Habana. Disponible en http//elibros.mes.edu.cu

Alcántara J. M. (2000): *Comportamiento reproductivo histórico y actual de un rebaño de hembras.* Siboney de Cuba perteneciente a la Empresa Pecuaria V Congreso Venegas. Orientador Científico Luis O. Alba. Trabajo de Curso. Sede Universitaria, Sancti Spíritus.

Álvarez, I., Capote, J., Traoré, A., Fonseca, N., Pérez, K., Cuervo, M., Fernández, I., Goyache, F. (2012): *Genetic relationships of the Cuban hair sheep inferred from microsatellite polymorphism. Small Ruminant Research.* 104:89-93.

Anónimo (1994): *Crianza del búfalo de agua. Elementos Básicos.* Grupo Nacional de Búfalos. Ciudad de La Habana.

Anónimo (2006): *Manual de Ganadería Vacuna*, Editado por el Ministerio de la Agricultura de Cuba. Cap. 3, pp 78.

Anónimo (2013): *Código Genético,* en EcuRed. Enciclopedia cubana.

Avendaño, L., Álvarez, F.D., Salomé, J., Correa, A., Molina, L., Cisneros, F. (2002): *Evaluación de algunos rasgos productivos del Borrego Pelibuey en el noroeste de México.* Resultados preliminares. Revista Cubana de Ciencia Agrícola. 38:131–136.

Barba, F. (1978): *Desarrollo testicular, producción y calidad seminal de los toros sementales Holstein x cebú en distintos grados de cruzamiento.* Tesis en Opción al grado científico de Ciencias Veterinarias. Universidad de Veterinaria de Brno, República Checa

Boichand, D., Grosh, C., Bourgeois, F. et al (2003): *Detection of genes influencing economic traits in three French dairy cattle breeds.* Genetics Selection Evolution 35:77-102.

Calzadilla, D., Soto, E., Hernández, M., González María Teresa et al. (2009): *Ganadería Tropical.* Editorial Félix Varela, La Habana, Cap. IX, pp 222.

Cantet, R.J., Gualdrón Duarte J.L., Munilla Leguizamón, S. (2008): *Selección genómica.* Revista Argentina de producción Animal 28(2):133-136.

Corzo, J., García, L., Silva, J., Pérez, E. (2009): *Zootecnia General. Un enfoque ecológico.* Ed. Félix Varela, La Habana. Cap. 2, pp. 36.

De la Loma J.L. (1963): *Genética General y Aplicada.* 3ra Ed. Unión Tipográfica Editorial Hispano Americana, Pp 365

Díaz, Oscar H. (1981): *Herencia y Fertilidad en Bovinos.* Impreso Graficinco, S.A, Madrid, pp.23.

Espinoza J., Palacios A., de Luna R., Ávila N., Guerra D., González – Peña D., et al. (2007): *Componentes de (co)varianza para caracteres de crecimiento y reproducción en ganado cebú en Cuba.* Arch Zootec 56(216):919-927.

Fernández J. y Tronco M.A (2011): *Influencia de factores no genéticos en la producción de leche del Siboney de Cuba.* Rev. Salud Anim.33(2):12-20.

Gallo, J.M. y Parrado O. (2015): *Genética y Mejoramiento Agropecuario.* Ed. Pueblo y Educación, La Habana. Cap II pp 55.

García S. y Planas Teresa (2003): *Manual de Crianza del Búfalo.* Ed. Sociedad cubana de criadores de búfalos. ACPA. Libro electrónico. Cap. 3, pp. 4.

Guitov, H. (2006): *Selección de Reproductores Bovinos.* 6ta Jornadas Nacionales Crías Bovinas Intensivas. 15-16 agosto, Venado-Tuerto, Santa Fe, Argentina

Hóly, L. y Barba, F. (1973): *Desarrollo y valores testimétricos de los toros de las razas B. Swiss y Holstein en el clima subtropical.* Rev. Cubana de Inseminación Artificial, La Habana, julio-agosto, 4-14,

Homedes J. y Haro-García F. (1966): *Zoogenética.* Empresa Consolidada de Artes Gráficas. Habana. Cap. 3 pp 581.

Lasley John F. (1973): *Genetics of Livestock Improvement.* Ed. Instituto Cubano del Libro, La Habana. Cap. 12, pp 94.

López, Delia. (2000): *Evaluación de los cruzamientos en las ganaderías de doble propósito. Su desarrollo en Cuba.* I Congreso Internacional sobre mejoramiento Animal, del 3 al 5 de mayo. Palacio de las Convenciones. La Habana.

Planas, Teresa. (1994): *Lechería de Búfalos. Una gota de mi ciudad al desarrollo ganadero.* Rvta ACPA 2: 40-45.

Planas Teresa, Rico Carmen, Ribas Miriam, Pérez Tania et al. (2002): *La Genética en Manos del Criador.* Libro electrónico en PDF. ACPA, Cuba.

Pulgarón P. y Pascual Carmen (1997): *Manual de Genética y Mejora Animal.* Editorial Pueblo y Educación. Cap. 4 pp 67.

Meirelles, S., Espasandin A., Mattar M., de Queiroz S. (2009): *Genetic and environmental effects on sexual precocity traits in Nellore cattle.* R Bras Zootec 38(8):1488-1493.

Meuwissen, T.H., Hayes, B., and Goddard, M.E. (2001): *Prediction of total genetic value using genomewide dense marker maps.* Genetics 157: 1819-1829.

Montes Ineida. (1995): *Aspectos reproductivos del macho cebú cubano.* Centro de Investigaciones para el Mejoramiento Animal (CIMA), Cuba.

Morrys L., Tyner P., Morris L., Forgason L., Williams S., Young F. (1989): *Correlation of testicular circumference and age in American Brahman bulls.* Theriologenology 31:489-494.

NRAG 212 (2012): *Patrón de la raza Cebú cubano e identificación obligatoria.* Editado por CENCOP. MINAG. Cuba

NRAG 232 (2011): *Patrón de la raza Holstein e identificación obligatoria.* Editado por CENCOP. MINAG. Cuba

NRAG 234 (2011): *Patrón de la raza Suiza Parda e identificación obligatoria.* Editado por CENCOP. MINAG. Cuba

Saatchi, M., Ward, J, and Garrick, D.J. (2012): *Accuracies of direct genomic breeding values in Hereford beef cattle using national or international training populations.* Journal of Animal Science 91: 1538-1551.

Glossary

DNA: Deoxyribonucleic acid. It is the genetic material of living beings, which exists in the cell nucleus in the form of a double helix.

Allele: Particular form of a gene in a genetic locus of a chromosome. Alternative forms of a gene in the same locus; for example, two possible alleles in the v locus of barley are v and V. The term allele or allelomorph was coined by William Bateson; it literally means "alternative form".

RNA: Ribonucleic acid. It plays an active role in protein synthesis in three of its forms: messenger RNA, transfer RNA and ribosomal RNA.

Monoclonal antibody: Structurally identical antibodies that recognize only one type of antigen.

Autosome: Non-sexual chromosome. The human genome is made up of 22 pairs of autosomes and two sexual chromosomes.

Biotechnology: Any technology that uses living organisms or parts of organisms to make or modify products that improve plants or animals, or develop microorganisms for specific uses.

Character: Observable characteristic transmitted by genes. Example: coat color.

Karyotype: Photographic display of the number, shape and size of the chromosomes of an organism.

DNA chips: Miniaturized device, the size of a microscope slide, that contains thousands of printed DNA fragments. These fragments can represent the entire genome.

Genetic code: It is the set of rules that defines the translation of a nucleotide sequence in RNA into an amino acid sequence in a protein in all living beings. The code defines the relationship between sequences of three nucleotides, called codons, and amino acids. In this way, each codon corresponds to a specific amino acid.

Convexilinear: Zootechnics. Morphological type referring to the convex profile of animals or breeds. E.g. Zebu.

Cloning: The production of multiple copies of a cell or its DNA.

Homologous chromosomes: Chromosomes that pair during meiosis. They have the same length and position of the centromere, and share the same genes.

Microsatellite DNA: Short DNA sequences (fragments) that are found very repeated in certain regions of the genome of eukaryotic cells and whose function is currently unknown. The variations observed in the number of repetitions serve to differentiate two individuals of the same species.

Diploid: A complete set of chromosomes, half of which belongs to each parent.

Dominance: Genetic effects due to interactions between alleles within a locus. For example, when there is complete dominance, genotypes containing one or two copies of the dominant allele have the same phenotype.

Dominant: An allele whose effect is the same in homozygous and heterozygous conditions.

Genes: (from the Greek genos: birth) are specific segments of DNA (chromosome) responsible for a certain character. They are the functional unit of inheritance. A gene is considered to be the segment of the DNA molecule that contains the code for a particular protein.

Genome: The totality of genetic information possessed by a particular organism or species. In eukaryotic beings, the genome comprises the DNA contained in the nucleus, organized into chromosomes, and the mitochondrial genome. The term was coined in 1920 by Hans Winkler, professor of Botany at the University of Hamburg, Germany, as an acronym of the words gene and chromosome.

Genotyping: Genotyping, or genotyping or genetic characterization, is understood as the process of determining the genotype or genomic content, in the form of DNA, specific to a biological organism, through a laboratory procedure.

Heterozygous: Originates from the union of gametes that differ in the class, quantity or arrangement of their genes. It is generally used with respect to particular genetic differences.

Homozygous: Derived from the union of identical gametes with respect to the class, quantity and arrangement of their genes or part of them.

Immortality: When individuals in a population leave descendants maintaining their genotype from one generation to the next.

Locus: Position occupied by a gene in a chromosome in relation to its linear order. Plural loci.

Markers: Reference points on chromosomes that show traits of genetic variability. They are any molecular phenotype originating from a specific gene. They are DNA sequences or polymorphic proteins derived from a simple chromosomal location. If they comply with Mendel's basic laws of inheritance, they are Genetic Markers.

Mutations: Source of genetic variability in the population. They may or may not generate changes in the sequence of proteins that encode the genes and of course affect or not the functions of the organisms.

Progeny: 1- Caste, generation or family from which an animal originates or descends.

      2- Descendants or set of children of someone.

Genetic variability: This refers to the variation in the genetic material of a population or species and includes genomes. For natural selection to act on a trait, there must be something to select for, i.e. several alleles for the gene encoding that trait. Furthermore, the more variation there is, the more evolution there is.

Author's review

The author Luis Orlando Alba Gómez, PhD, Full Professor, Expert in Bovine Reproduction. Former Head of the Animal Reproduction Department for 50 years at the Universidad Central de L.V. and José Martí in Sancti Spiritus, Cuba. He has directed more than 30 Diploma Theses, 15 Specialization Theses and two PhDs in Veterinary Sciences. He has published 28 articles in journals and five scientific books.

a

b

www.ingramcontent.com/pod-product-compliance
Lightning Source LLC
Chambersburg PA
CBHW052252220526
45471CB00001B/307